KARBVELOUS KETO

Transform your Plate, Transform Your Life
Christmas Sweets Edition

Carolyn Boheler, PhD

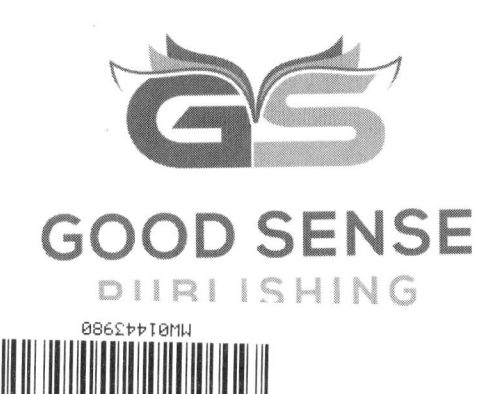

GOOD SENSE PUBLISHING

Copyright © 2024 by Carolyn Boheler

All rights reserved. No part of this book may be used or reproduced in any form whatsoever without written permission.

Printed in the United States of America.

For more information, or to book an event, contact :

info@GoodSensePublishing.com
https://GoodSensePublishing.com

Book design by Good Sense Publishing
Cover design by Good Sense Publishing

First Edition: November 2024

KARBVELOUS KETO I

INTRODUCTION A KETO CHRISTMAS TO REMEMBER 6

TIPS AND TRICKS FOR KETO CHRISTMAS CANDY 8

VIRTA –ONLINE COMMUNITY 11

CHOCOLATE CHIP PECAN SNOWBALLS....................................12

SINCKERDOODLES 13

LINZER COOKIES 16

PECAN PIE BARS 18

CRANBERRY CHEESECAKE 20

BUTTERY SHORTBREAD COOKIES 24

CHOCOLATE COVERED CHERRIES 26

KETO MOUNDS BARS..28

KETO PEPPERMINT BARK 30

KETO CHOCOLATE COVERED CARAMELS 32

CHOCOLATE TRUFFLES 35

CHOCOLATE COCONUT HAYSTACKS 36

SPICED NUTS 38

KETO NUT BRITTLE 40

PECAN CLUSTERS..42

MAPLE WALNUT FUDGE 44

KETO ALMOND ROCA 46

KETO CANDY CANE FAT BOMBS 50

KETO MARSHMALLOWS 52

KETO HOLIDAY GUMMY BEARS 56

WHITE CHOCOLATE PEPPERMINT BARK..............................58

CLASSIC CHOCOLATE FUDGE	60
CRANBERRY PISTACHIO BARK	62
PEANUT BUTTER FUDGE	64
LAYERED PEPPERMINT FUDGE	66
SALTED KETO CARAMELS	68
HOLIDAY TAFFY	70
GINGERBREAD CARAMEL CHEWS	72
COCONUT MACADAMIA CARAMELS	74
HOT COCOA FAT BOMBS	76
EGGNOG FAT BOMBS	78
PEPPERMINT MOCHA FAT BOMBS	80
CINNAMON ROLL FAT BOMBS	82
SUGAR FREE SWEETENERS	84
KETO CANDY MAKING TIPS	90
STORAGE & SHELF LIFE OF KETO CANDIES	95
GIFT WRAPPING IDEAS	100
CONCLUSION	106
ABOUT THE AUTHOR	107
BOOKS BY MY MOTHER	110
ACKNOWLEDGMENTS	111

Introduction: A Keto Christmas To Remember

The holiday season is a time of joy, togetherness, and cherished traditions. And for many of us, these traditions are woven with the delicious aromas of Christmas candies, cookies, and sweets that bring warmth and comfort to our gatherings. But if you're living a keto lifestyle, you may have felt a pang of concern as you face the holiday spread. How can you enjoy Christmas without the sugar-laden treats that tempt you at every turn?

"Karbvelous Keto, Christmas Sweets Edition" was created to answer that question—and so much more. In this cookbook, we've reinvented holiday classics with a keto twist, bringing you the best of Christmas flavors and textures without the carb overload. Think creamy peppermint bark, rich chocolate fudge, crispy spiced nuts, and buttery shortbread cookies—all reimagined to fit your keto goals. These recipes will let you indulge in your favorite sweets without the guilt, offering the taste of tradition in a way that aligns with your health journey.

As a longtime advocate of the keto lifestyle, I know the challenges that come with navigating the holidays on a low-carb diet. But I also know the rewards: reduced inflammation, steady energy, and the peace of mind that comes from nourishing your body well. With these recipes, I've crafted a collection of keto-friendly sweets that will help you stay on track without sacrificing flavor or festive cheer.

This cookbook goes beyond recipes, too. You'll find practical tips for swapping out sugar, using keto-friendly flours, and selecting holiday-friendly spices that bring warmth and comfort to each bite. Whether you're making treats for family, friends, or just yourself, these keto-friendly sweets are sure to bring smiles and spread joy without derailing your progress.

So, as you prepare for a season of celebrations, remember that the spirit of Christmas isn't about deprivation. It's about savoring the moments, cherishing loved ones, and making memories—one delicious, keto-friendly bite at a time. May this book inspire you to enjoy every holiday treat while staying true to your health goals, letting you experience all the sweetness of Christmas without any of the sugar.

Here's to a *Karbvelous* Keto Christmas—may it be as joyful, satisfying, and magical as ever!

I am not a medical doctor, and nothing in this book should be taken as medical advice. It's essential to consult with your own doctor before beginning any diet or lifestyle change to ensure it's safe and suitable for you. My background is not in the medical field; my doctorate is in metaphysics and religion. This book is intended to offer insights and ideas based on my personal experience and research but should never replace professional medical guidance.

I've included links to items found on Amazon that are used in the recipes within this book. When you click one of these links, I may earn a small commission, but rest assured, your price will not be higher because of it. Occasionally, you might even find a better deal!

The links are clickable on the kindle or ebook versions, or you can find a page of links at www.GoodSensePublishing.

Tips and Tricks For Keto Christmas Candy

Christmas is a season for celebration, and what would the holidays be without festive treats? Sticking to a keto lifestyle doesn't mean missing out on the joy of indulging in holiday sweets. With a few tweaks and smart substitutions, you can enjoy your favorite holiday treats without the carb overload. Here are some tips and tricks to help you savor every moment this Christmas while staying true to your keto goals.

Choose The Right Sweeteners

The key to keto-friendly candy is using sugar alternatives that won't spike blood sugar. For homemade treats, opt for natural sweeteners like:

- Erythritol: This sugar alcohol doesn't affect blood glucose levels, making it a great choice for keto sweets.
- Monk Fruit: A natural, zero-carb sweetener that works well in recipes needing that "sugar" taste.
- Stevia: A plant-derived sweetener that's versatile and pairs well with chocolate and peppermint flavors.
- Allulose: Known for its clean taste and ability to caramelize, allulose is a great choice for fudge or toffee.

Go Dark With Chocolate

Milk chocolate is high in sugar, but dark chocolate can be a great keto-friendly option. Look for chocolate that is 85% cacao or higher, or seek out **sugar-free chocolate** sweetened with stevia or erythritol. You can use these for all your Christmas classics—think keto Mounds bars, peppermint bark, or even chocolate-dipped pecans.

Add a Festive Touch with Flavor Extracts

Essences like peppermint, almond, and vanilla add that holiday magic without carbs. Peppermint extract brings a burst of Christmas flavor to candies like keto bark, and a drop or two of almond or vanilla extract can give a classic holiday richness to your sweets without any added sugar.

Incorporate Nuts and Seeds

Nuts like almonds, pecans, and walnuts add texture, flavor, and healthy fats to keto Christmas candies. Use them whole in chocolate barks or chop them for a bit of crunch in fudge and fat bombs. They're not only delicious but also packed with nutrients that keep you feeling satisfied longer.

Use Coconut in Creative Ways

Unsweetened shredded coconut, coconut oil, and coconut cream are fantastic ingredients for keto-friendly treats. Coconut oil can add a smooth, creamy texture to fudge or chocolate treats, while shredded coconut brings the right texture to recreate favorites like Mounds bars.

Experiment with Coconut or Almond Flour

When making holiday cookies, a bit of almond or coconut flour can go a long way. These low-carb flours provide a similar texture to traditional flours, letting you enjoy keto-friendly sugar cookies, peppermint chocolate cookies, and other holiday classics.

Keep Portions in Mind

Even with keto-friendly ingredients, holiday treats are best enjoyed in moderation. It can be easy to overindulge, especially with homemade goodies. Portioning out your sweets ahead of time can help you stay on track and enjoy them mindfully.

Remember Fat Bombs for Quick Treats

Fat bombs are a keto staple because they're easy to make and can be flavored to suit the season. Peppermint mocha, chocolate peanut butter, and vanilla-almond are great flavors for Christmas-themed fat bombs. You can even dress them up by rolling them in chopped nuts, shredded coconut, or cocoa powder.

Plan Ahead with Keto Friendly Swaps

If you know you'll be attending holiday gatherings or hosting family, prepare a few of your favorite keto-friendly treats in advance. This way, you'll always have an option on hand that satisfies your cravings without derailing your diet. Having treats like keto fudge or peppermint bark ready will help you avoid the temptation of traditional sugary sweets.

Focus on Flavor – Not Sugar

Christmas treats are all about rich flavors and comforting textures, not just sweetness. Play up spices like cinnamon, ginger, and nutmeg, which are naturally low in carbs and bring a cozy, holiday warmth to your dishes.

By following these tips, you can enjoy the season's best flavors without sacrificing your keto lifestyle. This Christmas, let the joy be in both the taste of your treats and the peace of mind knowing they're as keto-friendly as they are festive!

Let me know if you'd like to add more specific recipes or preparation tips!

Virta – Online Community

With the help of the Virta community, I was able to lose a significant amount of inflammation, which directly led to noticeable weight loss. This community became my lifeline, providing accountability and constant encouragement on my ketogenic journey. From sharing delicious, low-carb recipes to offering practical tips and tricks, the Virta community was there every step of the way. Together, we tackled meal planning, managed cravings, and celebrated each success. The support I received truly made the ketogenic lifestyle easier and more enjoyable, helping me achieve sustainable health and weight-loss results.

Finding Virta online was a game-changer! Their straightforward application process makes it easy to start, and many insurance plans now cover Virta's services, making this powerful support system accessible to many people. Once you're in, Virta equips you with all the essentials for a successful journey: a high-quality weight scale, a food scale, and tools to track blood glucose and ketone levels. They also provide books filled with recipes, practical guidelines, and valuable tips to help you stay on track. With Virta, you're fully supported and ready to dive into your health goals with confidence!

Chocolate Chip Pecan Snowballs

Ingredients:

- 1 cup almond flour
- 1/2 cup finely chopped pecans
- 1/4 cup butter, softened
- 1/4 cup powdered erythritol (or another keto-friendly powdered sweetener)
- 1/2 tsp vanilla extract
- 1/4 cup sugar-free chocolate chips
- Additional powdered erythritol for dusting

Instructions:

1. Preheat oven to 350°F (175°C). Line a baking sheet with parchment paper.
2. In a medium mixing bowl, combine almond flour, softened butter, powdered erythritol, and vanilla extract. Mix until smooth.
3. Fold in the chopped pecans and chocolate chips.
4. Roll the dough into 1-inch balls and place them on the prepared baking sheet.
5. Bake for 10-12 minutes or until the edges are lightly golden. Remove from the oven and let them cool completely on the baking sheet (they will firm up as they cool).
6. Once cooled, dust with additional powdered erythritol for a snowy effect.

Nutritional Information (per cookie, assuming 20 cookies):

- **Calories:** 75
- **Fat:** 7g
- **Protein:** 1.5g
- **Total Carbs:** 3g
- **Fiber:** 1g
- **Net Carbs:** 2g

Enjoy these delicious, buttery, melt-in-your-mouth cookies guilt-free! They're perfect for satisfying a sweet tooth without breaking keto.

Sinckerdoodles

Ingredients:

- 1 1/4 cups almond flour
- 1/4 cup coconut flour
- 1/4 cup butter, softened
- 1/4 cup powdered erythritol (or another keto-friendly powdered sweetener)
- 1 large egg
- 1 tsp vanilla extract
- 1/2 tsp baking powder
- 1/4 tsp cream of tartar
- Pinch of salt

Cinnomon Sugar Coating:

- 2 tbsp erythritol (granulated or powdered, based on preference)
- 1 tsp ground cinnamon

Instructions:

1. Preheat the oven to 350°F (175°C) and line a baking sheet with parchment paper.
2. In a medium mixing bowl, cream together the softened butter and powdered erythritol until smooth.
3. Add the egg and vanilla extract, and mix until well combined.
4. In a separate bowl, whisk together almond flour, coconut flour, baking powder, cream of tartar, and salt. Gradually add the dry ingredients to the wet ingredients, mixing until a soft dough forms.
5. In a small bowl, combine the erythritol and cinnamon for the coating.
6. Roll the dough into 1-inch balls, then roll each ball in the cinnamon-sugar mixture.
7. Place the balls on the prepared baking sheet and slightly flatten them with your fingers or the back of a spoon.

8. Bake for 8-10 minutes, until the edges are golden. Allow the cookies to cool on the baking sheet before transferring them to a wire rack.

Nutritional Information (per cookie, assuming 18 cookies)

- **Calories:** 65
- **Fat:** 6g
- **Protein:** 1.5g
- **Total Carbs:** 2.5g
- **Fiber:** 1g
- **Net Carbs:** 1.5g

These snickerdoodles are delightfully soft with a perfect cinnamon-sugar coating, bringing a cozy flavor without the carbs!

Linzer Cookies

Ingredients:

- 1 1/2 cups almond flour
- 1/4 cup coconut flour
- 1/2 cup butter, softened
- 1/3 cup powdered erythritol (or another keto-friendly powdered sweetener)
- 1 large egg
- 1 tsp vanilla extract
- 1/4 tsp salt
- 1/4 tsp baking powder
- 1/4 cup sugar-free raspberry or strawberry jam

Instructions:

1. In a large mixing bowl, cream together the softened butter and powdered erythritol until light and fluffy.
2. Add the egg and vanilla extract, and mix until well combined.
3. In a separate bowl, whisk together almond flour, coconut flour, salt, and baking powder.
4. Gradually add the dry ingredients to the wet ingredients, mixing until a soft dough forms.
5. Divide the dough in half, shape into discs, wrap in plastic wrap, and chill for at least 30 minutes.
6. Preheat the oven to 350°F (175°C) and line a baking sheet with parchment paper.
7. Roll out each dough disc between two sheets of parchment paper to about 1/8-inch thickness.
8. Use a round cookie cutter (about 2 inches) to cut out circles. In half of the cookies, cut out a small shape (like a heart or star) from the center to create a "window" for the top of the Linzer cookie.
9. Carefully transfer the cookies to the prepared baking sheet.
10. Bake for 10-12 minutes, or until edges are golden. Let them cool completely on the baking sheet.

11. Once cooled, spread a small amount of sugar-free jam on the flat side of each whole cookie. Top with a "window" cookie and press gently.
12. Optional: Dust with powdered erythritol for a snowy finish.

Nutritional Information (per cookie, assuming 16 cookies – 32 single cookies)

- **Calories:** 90
- **Fat:** 8g
- **Protein:** 2g
- **Total Carbs:** 4g
- **Fiber:** 2g
- **Net Carbs:** 2g

These Keto Linzer Cookies are buttery, nutty, and perfectly sweetened, making them a great choice for holiday baking or a festive treat!

Pecan Pie Bars

Ingredients

For the Crust:

- 1 1/2 cups almond flour
- 1/4 cup coconut flour
- 1/4 cup butter, melted
- 2 tbsp powdered erythritol (or another keto-friendly sweetener)
- 1/4 tsp salt

For the Pecan Filling:

- 3/4 cup pecans, roughly chopped
- 1/2 cup butter
- 1/3 cup sugar-free maple syrup
- 1/4 cup powdered erythritol
- 1 large egg
- 1 tsp vanilla extract
- 1/4 tsp salt

Instructions

1. **Preheat the oven** to 350°F (175°C). Line an 8x8-inch baking pan with parchment paper, leaving some overhang for easy removal.
2. **Make the Crust:**
    - In a medium mixing bowl, combine almond flour, coconut flour, melted butter, powdered erythritol, and salt. Mix until well combined.
    - Press the crust mixture evenly into the bottom of the prepared baking pan.
    - Bake for 10-12 minutes, or until the edges are lightly golden. Remove from the oven and let cool slightly.
3. **Prepare the Filling:**
    - In a saucepan over medium heat, melt the butter and stir in the sugar-free maple syrup, powdered

- erythritol, and salt. Let it simmer for 2-3 minutes, stirring occasionally.
    - Remove from heat and allow to cool slightly, then whisk in the egg and vanilla extract until smooth.
    - Stir in the chopped pecans.
4. **Assemble and Bake:**
    - Pour the pecan filling evenly over the pre-baked crust.
    - Return the pan to the oven and bake for an additional 20-25 minutes, or until the filling is set and the top is golden.
    - Let the bars cool completely in the pan, then lift them out using the parchment paper and slice into 16 squares.

Nutritional Information (per bar, assuming 16 bars):

- **Calories:** 150
- **Fat:** 14g
- **Protein:** 2g
- **Total Carbs:** 5g
- **Fiber:** 2g
- **Net Carbs:** 3g

These Keto Pecan Pie Bars are rich, buttery, and filled with all the nutty flavor you love, perfect for a low-carb dessert that won't derail your keto goals!

Cranberry Cheesecake

Ingredients:

For the Crust:

- 1 1/2 cups almond flour
- 1/4 cup melted butter
- 2 tbsp powdered erythritol
- 1/4 tsp salt

For the Cheesecake Filling:

- 3 (8 oz) packages cream cheese, softened
- 3/4 cup powdered erythritol
- 3 large eggs
- 1 tsp vanilla extract
- 1/2 cup sour cream
- 1 tbsp lemon juice

For the Cranberry Sauce Topping:

- 1 cup fresh or frozen cranberries
- 1/4 cup water
- 1/4 cup powdered erythritol
- 1/2 tsp vanilla extract
- 1/2 tsp lemon zest (optional)

Instructions:

Preheat the oven to 325°F (160°C). Grease a 9-inch springform pan and line the bottom with parchment paper.

1. **Make the Crust:**
    - In a medium bowl, mix almond flour, melted butter, powdered erythritol, and salt until combined.
    - Press the mixture evenly into the bottom of the prepared springform pan.
    - Bake for 10-12 minutes or until lightly golden. Set aside to cool.

2. **Prepare the Cheesecake Filling:**
    - In a large bowl, beat the softened cream cheese and powdered erythritol with an electric mixer until smooth and creamy.
    - Add the eggs, one at a time, mixing well after each addition.
    - Mix in the vanilla extract, sour cream, and lemon juice until fully incorporated.
    - Pour the cheesecake filling over the cooled crust, smoothing the top with a spatula.
3. **Bake the Cheesecake:**
    - Place the springform pan on a baking sheet and bake for 50-60 minutes, or until the center is set but slightly jiggly. Turn off the oven, crack the oven door, and allow the cheesecake to cool slowly for 1 hour.
    - Remove from the oven and let the cheesecake cool completely before refrigerating for at least 4 hours (or overnight for best results).
4. **Make the Cranberry Sauce Topping:**
    - In a small saucepan, combine the cranberries, water, and powdered erythritol. Bring to a simmer over medium heat and cook for 5-7 minutes, or until the cranberries soften and begin to burst.
    - Remove from heat and stir in the vanilla extract and lemon zest, if using. Allow the sauce to cool completely.
5. **Assemble:**
    - Once the cheesecake is fully chilled, spoon the cranberry sauce over the top, spreading it evenly.
    - Slice and serve.

Nutritional Information (per slice, assuming 12 slices)

- **Calories:** 230
- **Fat:** 21g
- **Protein:** 5g
- **Total Carbs:** 6g
- **Fiber:** 2g
- **Net Carbs:** 4g

Buttery Shortbread Cookies

These buttery, crumbly shortbread cookies are simple to make with just a few ingredients and are perfect for low-carb snacking or holiday treats.

Ingredients:

- 1 cup almond flour
- 1/4 cup coconut flour
- 1/2 cup unsalted butter, softened
- 1/4 cup powdered erythritol (or your preferred keto-friendly sweetener)
- 1 teaspoon vanilla extract
- 1/4 teaspoon salt

Instructions:

1. **Preheat the Oven:**
   - Preheat your oven to 350°F (175°C) and line a baking sheet with parchment paper.
2. **Prepare the Dough:**
   - In a mixing bowl, beat the softened butter and powdered erythritol until light and fluffy.
   - Add the vanilla extract and salt, mixing until well combined.
   - Gradually add the almond flour and coconut flour, stirring until the dough forms. The dough should be soft but not sticky.
3. **Shape the Cookies:**
   - Roll the dough into small balls (about 1 tablespoon each) and place them on the prepared baking sheet. Flatten each ball slightly with your hand or the back of a fork to form a cookie shape.
4. **Bake:**
   - Bake in the preheated oven for 10–12 minutes, or until the edges are golden brown.
   - Remove from the oven and let the cookies cool on the baking sheet for 5–10 minutes to firm up, then transfer to a wire rack to cool completely.

5. **Store and Serve:**
    - Store the cookies in an airtight container at room temperature for up to one week or in the fridge for up to two weeks.

Nutritional Information (per cookie, assuming 12 cookies)

- **Calories:** 100
- **Fat:** 9g
- **Protein:** 2g
- **Total Carbohydrates:** 3g
- **Fiber:** 1g
- **Net Carbs:** 2g

These Keto Buttery Shortbread Cookies are crumbly, buttery, and deliciously low in carbs. Enjoy them as a snack, dessert, or holiday treat!

Chocolate Covered Cherries

These chocolate-covered cherries are a delightful mix of juicy, sweet, and chocolatey, perfect for a low-carb holiday treat or an everyday indulgence.

Ingredients:

- 12 frozen pitted black cherries (look for unsweetened, or freeze fresh ones)
- 1/2 cup sugar-free dark chocolate chips (85% cacao or higher)
- 1 tablespoon coconut oil
- Optional: 1–2 drops liquid stevia or monk fruit sweetener (if you prefer a slightly sweeter chocolate coating)

Instructions:

1. **Prepare the Cherries:**
    - If using fresh cherries, wash and pit them, then freeze them on a baking sheet lined with parchment paper until firm. This helps the chocolate coating set quickly when dipped.
2. **Melt the Chocolate:**
    - In a microwave-safe bowl, combine the sugar-free dark chocolate chips and coconut oil. Microwave in 20-second intervals, stirring between each, until the chocolate is fully melted and smooth.

- If you want a slightly sweeter coating, add 1–2 drops of liquid stevia or monk fruit sweetener to the chocolate and stir well.
3. **Dip the Cherries:**
    - Using a fork or toothpick, dip each frozen cherry into the melted chocolate, ensuring it's fully coated.
    - Lift the cherry out, let the excess chocolate drip off, and place it on a parchment-lined baking sheet.
4. **Chill and Set:**
    - Place the chocolate-covered cherries in the fridge for about 15 minutes or until the chocolate has hardened.
5. **Store and Serve:**
    - Store the chocolate-covered cherries in an airtight container in the fridge for up to one week. Enjoy them cold for a refreshing, chocolatey treat!

Nutritional Information (per chocolate-covered cherry, assuming 12 serving):

- **Calories:** 35
- **Fat:** 3g
- **Protein:** 0.5g
- **Total Carbohydrates:** 2g
- **Fiber:** 1g
- **Net Carbs:** 1g

These Keto Chocolate-Covered Cherries are a delicious, guilt-free treat that combines juicy cherries with a rich, sugar-free chocolate coating. Perfect for low-carb snacking or sharing with friends!

Keto Mounds Bars

These keto Mounds bars are a low-carb take on the classic, combining creamy coconut filling with a rich chocolate coating. Perfect for satisfying your sweet cravings without compromising your keto lifestyle!

Ingredients:

For the Coconut Filling:

- 1 ½ cups unsweetened shredded coconut
- ½ cup coconut cream (or thick part of a can of coconut milk)
- ¼ cup powdered erythritol (or your preferred keto sweetener)
- 1 teaspoon vanilla extract

For the Chocolate Coating:

- 1 cup sugar-free dark chocolate chips (85% cacao or higher)
- 1 tablespoon coconut oil

Instructions:

1. **Prepare the Coconut Filling:**
   - In a bowl, mix together the shredded coconut, coconut cream, powdered erythritol, and vanilla extract until fully combined and sticky.
   - Shape the mixture into small rectangular bars (around 2 inches long).
   - Place the bars on a baking sheet lined with parchment paper and freeze for 30 minutes to set.
2. **Melt the Chocolate:**
   - In a microwave-safe bowl, melt the sugar-free chocolate chips and coconut oil in 20-second intervals, stirring between each until smooth.

3. **Coat the Bars:**
   - Remove the coconut bars from the freezer. Dip each bar in the melted chocolate using a fork, allowing any excess chocolate to drip off.
   - Place the coated bars back on the parchment-lined sheet and return them to the freezer for 10–15 minutes, or until the chocolate has hardened.
4. **Serve and Store:**
   - Once the bars are set, store them in an airtight container in the fridge for up to two weeks or in the freezer for up to three months.

Nutritional Information (per bar, assuming 10 bars)

- **Calories:** 130
- **Fat:** 12g
- **Protein:** 1g
- **Total Carbohydrates:** 5g
- **Fiber:** 3g
- **Net Carbs:** 2g

Enjoy your homemade keto Mounds bars guilt-free! They're rich, satisfying, and just sweet enough to keep your holiday season low in carbs and high in flavor.

Keto Peppermint Bark

This low-carb peppermint bark combines creamy white and dark chocolate layers with a hint of peppermint and a satisfying crunch. It's easy to make and only takes a few minutes to set!

Ingredients:

- 1 cup sugar-free dark chocolate chips (85% cacao or higher)
- 1 cup sugar-free white chocolate chips
- 2 tablespoons coconut oil, divided
- 1/2 teaspoon peppermint extract
- 1–2 tablespoons crushed sugar-free peppermint candies or sugar-free peppermint sticks (optional, for topping)

Instructions:

1. **Prepare the Dark Chocolate Layer:**
   - In a microwave-safe bowl, melt the sugar-free dark chocolate chips with 1 tablespoon of coconut oil in 20-second intervals, stirring in between, until smooth.
   - Stir in 1/4 teaspoon of peppermint extract.
   - Pour the melted chocolate onto a parchment-lined baking sheet and spread it into an even layer, about 1/4 inch thick.
   - Place the baking sheet in the freezer for about 10 minutes, or until the chocolate is firm.

2. **Prepare the White Chocolate Layer:**
    - In a separate bowl, melt the sugar-free white chocolate chips with the remaining tablespoon of coconut oil in 20-second intervals, stirring until smooth.
    - Stir in the remaining 1/4 teaspoon of peppermint extract.
    - Pour the melted white chocolate over the firm dark chocolate layer and spread evenly.
3. **Add the Peppermint Crunch:**
    - If using, sprinkle the crushed sugar-free peppermint candies over the top while the white chocolate is still soft.
4. **Set the Bark:**
    - Return the baking sheet to the freezer for 15–20 minutes, or until completely set.
    - Once firm, break the bark into pieces and store it in an airtight container in the fridge for up to two weeks.

Nutritional Information (per serving, assuming 12 servings)

- **Calories:** 110
- **Fat:** 9g
- **Protein:** 1g
- **Total Carbohydrates:** 5g
- **Fiber:** 3g
- **Net Carbs:** 2g

This keto peppermint bark brings all the minty-chocolate goodness of traditional bark with a fraction of the carbs. It's a perfect holiday treat to share with family and friends—or keep for yourself! Enjoy!

Keto Chocolate Covered Caramels

These chocolate-covered caramels are rich, chewy, and perfectly sweetened for a keto-friendly treat. You'll love how easy they are to make, and they're perfect for holiday gatherings or gifting!

Ingredients:

For the Caramel:

- 1/2 cup unsalted butter
- 1/2 cup heavy cream
- 1/4 cup powdered erythritol (or preferred keto-friendly sweetener)
- 1/2 teaspoon vanilla extract
- Pinch of salt

For the Chocolate Coating:

- 1 cup sugar-free dark chocolate chips (85% cacao or higher)
- 1 tablespoon coconut oil

Instructions:

1. **Make the Caramel:**
   - In a medium saucepan over medium heat, melt the butter and allow it to brown slightly, stirring constantly. This should take about 5 minutes, and the butter will develop a nutty aroma.
   - Once browned, reduce the heat to low and add the heavy cream, powdered erythritol, and salt. Stir well to combine.
   - Continue to cook the mixture on low heat, stirring frequently, until it thickens and turns a rich caramel color, about 8–10 minutes.
   - Remove the saucepan from heat, stir in the vanilla extract, and let the caramel cool slightly before pouring it into a parchment-lined dish.
   - Place the caramel in the fridge for 1–2 hours to set, then cut into small squares once firm.

2. **Coat the Caramels in Chocolate:**
    - In a microwave-safe bowl, melt the sugar-free chocolate chips with the coconut oil in 20-second intervals, stirring until smooth.
    - Using a fork, dip each caramel square into the melted chocolate, letting the excess drip off before placing it on a parchment-lined tray.
    - Place the tray in the fridge for about 15 minutes, or until the chocolate has fully set.
3. **Serve and Store:**
    - Store the chocolate-covered caramels in an airtight container in the fridge for up to two weeks.

Nutritional Information (per caramel, assuming 16 pieces)

- **Calories:** 90
- **Fat:** 9g
- **Protein:** 0.5g
- **Total Carbohydrates:** 5g
- **Fiber:** 3g
- **Net Carbs:** 2g

Enjoy these keto chocolate-covered caramels guilt-free! They're perfect for satisfying a sweet tooth while keeping carbs low.

Chocolate Truffles

These smooth, creamy truffles are made with rich chocolate, heavy cream, and a touch of vanilla, creating a luxurious bite-sized treat with minimal carbs.

Ingredients:

- 1 cup sugar-free dark chocolate chips (85% cacao or higher)
- 1/2 cup heavy cream
- 2 tablespoons unsalted butter
- 1 teaspoon vanilla extract
- 1 tablespoon powdered erythritol (or your preferred keto sweetener, optional for added sweetness)
- **Optional Coatings:** cocoa powder, finely chopped nuts, shredded coconut, or powdered erythritol

Instructions:

1. **Melt the Chocolate:**
    - Place the chocolate chips and butter in a heatproof bowl.
    - In a small saucepan over medium heat, bring the heavy cream just to a simmer (do not let it boil). Pour the hot cream over the chocolate and butter.
    - Let the mixture sit for about 1–2 minutes to melt the chocolate, then stir until smooth and fully combined.
2. **Add Flavoring:**
    - Stir in the vanilla extract and powdered erythritol, if using, until well incorporated.
3. **Chill the Mixture:**
    - Cover the bowl and refrigerate for 1–2 hours, or until the chocolate mixture is firm enough to scoop.
4. **Shape the Truffles:**
    - Using a small spoon or a melon baller, scoop out the chilled chocolate mixture and roll it into small balls (about 1 inch in diameter) with your hands.

5. **Coat the Truffles:**
    - Roll each truffle in your desired coating, such as cocoa powder, finely chopped nuts, shredded coconut, or powdered erythritol.
6. **Serve and Store:**
    - Store the truffles in an airtight container in the fridge for up to two weeks.

Nutritional Information:

- **Calories:** 80
- **Fat:** 8g
- **Protein:** 1g
- **Total Carbohydrates:** 4g
- **Fiber:** 2g
- **Net Carbs:** 2g

These keto truffles are a rich, indulgent treat that melts in your mouth, perfect for satisfying chocolate cravings without the carb guilt. Enjoy!

Chocolate Coconut Haystacks

These crunchy, chocolatey haystacks combine shredded coconut, nuts, and sugar-free chocolate for a satisfying low-carb treat.

Ingredients:

- 1 cup unsweetened shredded coconut
- 1/2 cup slivered or chopped almonds (or other nuts, like pecans or walnuts)
- 1/2 cup sugar-free dark chocolate chips (85% cacao or higher)
- 2 tablespoons coconut oil
- Optional: 1 tablespoon powdered erythritol (or preferred keto-friendly sweetener) for a touch of added sweetness
- 1/2 teaspoon vanilla extract

Instructions:

1. **Toast the Coconut and Nuts (Optional):**
   - In a dry skillet over medium heat, toast the shredded coconut and almonds for 3–5 minutes, stirring frequently, until golden and fragrant. This step is optional but adds extra flavor and crunch.
   - Set aside to cool.
2. **Melt the Chocolate:**
   - In a microwave-safe bowl, combine the sugar-free dark chocolate chips and coconut oil. Microwave in 20-second intervals, stirring between each, until smooth and fully melted.
   - Stir in the powdered erythritol, if using, and vanilla extract.
3. **Mix Ingredients:**
   - In a large bowl, combine the toasted coconut and almonds with the melted chocolate mixture. Stir well to ensure everything is coated in chocolate.
4. **Form the Haystacks:**
   - Line a baking sheet with parchment paper. Spoon small mounds of the mixture (about 1 tablespoon each) onto the sheet, shaping them into "haystacks."

5. **Chill and Set:**
   - Place the baking sheet in the fridge for about 20–30 minutes, or until the haystacks are firm and set.
6. **Store and Serve:**
   - Store the haystacks in an airtight container in the fridge for up to two weeks or in the freezer for longer storage. Enjoy them chilled for a perfect, crunchy keto treat!

Nutritional Information (per haystack, assuming 12 servings):

- **Calories:** 90
- **Fat:** 8g
- **Protein:** 1g
- **Total Carbohydrates:** 3g
- **Fiber:** 2g
- **Net Carbs:** 1g

These Keto Haystacks are the perfect combination of chocolate and crunch, with minimal carbs and maximum flavor. They're great for satisfying sweet cravings without the guilt!

Spiced Nuts

This mix of nuts is coated in butter, sweetener, and a blend of warm spices, making them a perfect keto-friendly treat for any occasion.

Ingredients:

- 1 cup raw almonds
- 1 cup raw pecans
- 1 cup raw walnuts
- 2 tablespoons unsalted butter, melted
- 2 tablespoons powdered erythritol (or your preferred keto-friendly sweetener)
- 1 teaspoon cinnamon
- 1/2 teaspoon nutmeg
- 1/4 teaspoon ground cloves
- 1/4 teaspoon cayenne pepper (optional, for a touch of heat)
- 1/2 teaspoon sea salt
- 1 teaspoon vanilla extract

Instructions:

1. **Preheat the Oven:**
   - Preheat your oven to 300°F (150°C). Line a baking sheet with parchment paper.
2. **Prepare the Spice Mixture:**
   - In a large bowl, combine the melted butter, powdered erythritol, cinnamon, nutmeg, cloves, cayenne pepper (if using), salt, and vanilla extract. Stir until well mixed.
3. **Coat the Nuts:**
   - Add the almonds, pecans, and walnuts to the bowl with the spice mixture. Toss well until the nuts are evenly coated.
4. **Bake the Nuts:**
   - Spread the coated nuts in a single layer on the prepared baking sheet. Bake for 20–25 minutes, stirring halfway through, until the nuts are toasted and fragrant.

5. **Cool and Serve:**
    - Remove from the oven and let the nuts cool completely. They will crisp up as they cool. Store in an airtight container at room temperature for up to two weeks.

Nutritional Information (per ¼ cup serving, about 10 servings total)

- **Calories:** 190
- **Fat:** 18g
- **Protein:** 4g
- **Total Carbohydrates:** 5g
- **Fiber:** 3g
- **Net Carbs:** 2g

These keto spiced nuts are perfect for a low-carb snack that's packed with flavor. Enjoy their crunch and warmth, whether it's a holiday gathering or just a cozy night in!

Keto Nut Brittle

This nut brittle is made with a blend of nuts and a keto-friendly caramel, creating a crispy, sweet treat that's perfect for snacking or gifting.

Ingredients:

- 1 cup mixed nuts (such as almonds, pecans, and walnuts)
- 1/2 cup powdered erythritol (or preferred keto-friendly sweetener)
- 1/4 cup unsalted butter
- 1/4 cup heavy cream
- 1/2 teaspoon vanilla extract
- 1/4 teaspoon salt
- Optional: 1/4 teaspoon cinnamon or pinch of cayenne for added warmth

Instructions:

1. **Prepare a Baking Sheet:**
    - Line a baking sheet with parchment paper or a silicone baking mat to prevent sticking.
2. **Toast the Nuts:**
    - Place the mixed nuts on the baking sheet and toast them in the oven at 350°F (175°C) for about 5 minutes, until they're lightly golden and fragrant. Set aside.

3. **Make the Caramel Sauce:**
   - In a medium saucepan over medium heat, melt the butter and add the powdered erythritol, stirring constantly.
   - Add the heavy cream and continue to stir until the mixture turns a golden brown color, about 4–6 minutes. Be careful not to burn it!
   - Remove the saucepan from heat and stir in the vanilla extract, salt, and any optional spices.
4. **Combine and Spread:**
   - Add the toasted nuts to the caramel mixture, stirring until they're fully coated.
   - Pour the nut mixture onto the prepared baking sheet, spreading it out into an even layer.
   - Let it cool completely at room temperature or pop it in the fridge to speed up the process.
5. **Break and Serve:**
   - Once hardened, break the nut brittle into pieces and enjoy!
   - Store in an airtight container at room temperature for up to two weeks.

Nutritional Information (per 1 oz piece, assuming 12 pieces)

- **Calories:** 120
- **Fat:** 11g
- **Protein:** 2g
- **Total Carbohydrates:** 4g
- **Fiber:** 2g
- **Net Carbs:** 2g

Enjoy this crunchy, keto-friendly nut brittle as a sweet, low-carb treat that's perfect for the holiday season!

Pecan Clusters

These pecan clusters are made with roasted pecans and sugar-free chocolate, creating a rich, crunchy treat that's low in carbs and high in flavor.

Ingredients:

- 1 cup pecan halves
- 1 cup sugar-free dark chocolate chips (85% cacao or higher)
- 1 tablespoon coconut oil (optional, for easier melting and smoother texture)

Instructions:

1. **Prepare the Pecans:**
    - Toast the pecan halves in a dry skillet over medium heat for 5–7 minutes, stirring frequently, until they're fragrant and lightly toasted. Set aside to cool slightly.
2. **Melt the Chocolate:**
    - In a microwave-safe bowl, combine the sugar-free chocolate chips and coconut oil. Microwave in 20-second intervals, stirring after each, until smooth and fully melted.
3. **Make the Clusters:**
    - Line a baking sheet with parchment paper.
    - Drop small clusters of pecans (about 3–4 halves per cluster) onto the baking sheet.
    - Spoon melted chocolate over each pecan cluster until well coated.
4. **Set the Clusters:**
    - Place the baking sheet in the fridge for 15–20 minutes, or until the chocolate has fully hardened.
5. **Serve and Store:**
    - Store the clusters in an airtight container in the fridge for up to two weeks.

Nutritional Information (per cluster, assuming 12 clusters)

- **Calories:** 90
- **Fat:** 9g
- **Protein:** 1g
- **Total Carbohydrates:** 4g
- **Fiber:** 2g
- **Net Carbs:** 2g

These keto pecan clusters are simple to make, perfectly sweetened, and satisfyingly crunchy. Enjoy them as a snack or dessert that keeps you on track with your low-carb goals!

Maple Walnut Fudge

This smooth, melt-in-your-mouth fudge is infused with maple flavor and studded with crunchy walnuts. It's quick to make and great for holiday gatherings or an anytime treat.

Ingredients:

- 1/2 cup unsalted butter
- 1/2 cup heavy cream
- 1/3 cup powdered erythritol (or preferred keto-friendly sweetener)
- 1/2 teaspoon maple extract
- 1/2 teaspoon vanilla extract
- 1/4 teaspoon salt
- 1/2 cup chopped walnuts

Instructions:

1. **Prepare the Fudge Mixture:**
    - In a medium saucepan over medium heat, melt the butter. Add the heavy cream and powdered erythritol, stirring constantly.
    - Continue to cook the mixture for about 8–10 minutes, stirring frequently, until it thickens and turns a light golden color. Be careful not to let it burn.
2. **Add Flavor and Nuts:**
    - Remove the saucepan from heat and stir in the maple extract, vanilla extract, and salt. Mix in the chopped walnuts.
3. **Set the Fudge:**
    - Line a small dish or pan (such as an 8x4-inch loaf pan) with parchment paper, leaving some overhang to make it easier to lift out the fudge later.
    - Pour the fudge mixture into the prepared pan, spreading it out evenly.
    - Refrigerate for at least 2 hours, or until fully set.
4. **Cut and Serve:**
    - Once set, lift the fudge out of the pan using the parchment paper and cut it into small squares.

5. **Store:**
    - Store the fudge in an airtight container in the fridge for up to two weeks.

Nutritional Information (per square, assuming 16 squares)

- **Calories:** 120
- **Fat:** 12g
- **Protein:** 1g
- **Total Carbohydrates:** 3g
- **Fiber:** 1g
- **Net Carbs:** 2g

This keto maple walnut fudge is creamy, nutty, and has the perfect hint of maple flavor. It's a wonderful low-carb treat that's easy to make and even easier to enjoy!

Keto Almond Roca

This crunchy, buttery toffee is topped with a layer of rich chocolate and a sprinkle of almonds, making it a delicious low-carb twist on the classic treat.

Ingredients:

For the Toffee:

- 1/2 cup unsalted butter
- 1/2 cup powdered erythritol (or preferred keto sweetener)
- 1/4 teaspoon vanilla extract
- 1/4 teaspoon salt
- 1/2 cup chopped almonds

For the Chocolate Coating:

- 1/2 cup sugar-free dark chocolate chips (85% cacao or higher)
- 1 teaspoon coconut oil (optional, for smoother melting)
- 1/4 cup finely chopped almonds (for dusting)

Instructions:

1. **Prepare the Toffee:**
   - In a medium saucepan over medium heat, melt the butter. Stir in the powdered erythritol and salt, cooking and stirring constantly.
   - Allow the mixture to come to a gentle boil. Continue cooking, stirring constantly, until the toffee reaches a golden brown color (around 300°F if using a candy thermometer), about 10 minutes. Be careful not to let it burn.
   - Remove the saucepan from heat and quickly stir in the vanilla extract and chopped almonds.
2. **Spread the Toffee:**
   - Line a baking sheet with parchment paper. Pour the hot toffee mixture onto the parchment, spreading it into an even layer about 1/4 inch thick.
   - Let the toffee cool slightly but not fully harden.
3. **Add the Chocolate Coating:**
   - In a microwave-safe bowl, melt the sugar-free chocolate chips and coconut oil in 20-second intervals, stirring until smooth.
   - Pour the melted chocolate over the toffee, spreading it into an even layer.
4. **Dust with Almonds:**
   - Sprinkle the finely chopped almonds over the melted chocolate.
5. **Set the Almond Roca:**
   - Let the toffee cool completely at room temperature or in the fridge until fully set.
   - Once set, break the Almond Roca into pieces.
6. **Store:**
   - Store the Almond Roca in an airtight container in the fridge for up to two weeks.

Nutritional Information (per piece, assuming 20 pieces):

- **Calories:** 90
- **Fat:** 9g
- **Protein:** 1g
- **Total Carbohydrates:** 4g
- **Fiber:** 2g
- **Net Carbs:** 2g

This keto Almond Roca is a delightful low-carb treat with a crunchy texture and rich flavor, perfect for holiday gifting or enjoying as a keto-friendly dessert!

Keto Candy Cane Fat Bombs

These peppermint fat bombs are perfect for satisfying your holiday sweet cravings while staying in ketosis. They're rich, creamy, and have a refreshing minty flavor!

Ingredients:

- 1/2 cup cream cheese, softened
- 1/4 cup unsalted butter, softened
- 1/4 cup coconut oil, softened
- 2–3 tablespoons powdered erythritol (or your preferred keto-friendly sweetener)
- 1/2 teaspoon peppermint extract
- Optional: red food coloring for a festive swirl
- Optional: 1–2 crushed sugar-free peppermint candies or sugar-free peppermint dust (for garnish)

Instructions:

1. **Prepare the Base:**
   - In a mixing bowl, combine the cream cheese, butter, and coconut oil. Mix until smooth and creamy.
2. **Add Flavoring:**
   - Add the powdered erythritol and peppermint extract. Mix thoroughly until all ingredients are well incorporated.
   - For a festive look, add a few drops of red food coloring and gently swirl it into the mixture with a knife to create a candy cane effect.
3. **Form the Fat Bombs:**
   - Scoop out small portions of the mixture (about 1 tablespoon each) and place them on a parchment-lined baking sheet. Shape into rounds if desired.
   - Optionally, sprinkle a little crushed sugar-free peppermint candy on top of each fat bomb for garnish.
4. **Set the Fat Bombs:**
   - Place the baking sheet in the freezer for about 30 minutes or until the fat bombs are firm.
5. **Serve and Store:**
   - Store the fat bombs in an airtight container in the fridge for up to one week or in the freezer for up to one month.

Nutrtional Information (per fat bomb, assuming 12 fat bombs)

- **Calories:** 80
- **Fat:** 8g
- **Protein:** 0.5g
- **Total Carbohydrates:** 1.5g
- **Fiber:** 0g
- **Net Carbs:** 1.5g

These Candy Cane Fat Bombs are perfect for holiday snacking or a quick, refreshing treat between meals. Enjoy the peppermint flavor and festive look without the carbs!

Keto Marshmallows

These marshmallows are light, fluffy, and have the classic marshmallow texture without the sugar. They're ideal for satisfying sweet cravings while keeping your carbs low.

Ingredients:

- 1 cup water, divided
- 3 tablespoons unflavored gelatin powder
- 1 cup powdered erythritol (or your preferred keto-friendly sweetener)
- 1/4 teaspoon salt
- 1 teaspoon vanilla extract

Instructions:

1. **Prepare the Gelatin:**
   - In the bowl of a stand mixer, add 1/2 cup of water. Sprinkle the gelatin powder over the water and let it sit for about 5 minutes to bloom.
2. **Make the Syrup:**
   - In a small saucepan, combine the remaining 1/2 cup of water, powdered erythritol, and salt. Heat over medium heat, stirring occasionally until the sweetener is fully dissolved and the mixture reaches a gentle simmer.
   - Remove the saucepan from heat.

3. **Combine and Whip:**
   - With the stand mixer on low speed, slowly pour the hot syrup mixture into the gelatin mixture.
   - Once combined, increase the mixer speed to high and whip for about 10–15 minutes, until the mixture has tripled in volume and is thick, fluffy, and glossy. Add the vanilla extract in the last minute of mixing.
4. **Set the Marshmallows:**
   - Line an 8x8-inch baking pan with parchment paper and lightly grease it with coconut oil or a non-stick spray.
   - Pour the marshmallow mixture into the prepared pan, spreading it evenly with a spatula.
   - Let the marshmallows sit at room temperature for at least 4 hours (or overnight) to fully set.
5. **Cut and Serve:**
   - Once set, remove the marshmallows from the pan and cut them into squares with a greased knife.
   - Optionally, you can dust the marshmallows with a little extra powdered erythritol to prevent sticking.
6. **Store:**
   - Store the marshmallows in an airtight container at room temperature for up to one week.

Nutritional Information (per marshmallow, assuming 16 marshmallows)

- **Calories:** 5
- **Fat:** 0g
- **Protein:** 1g
- **Total Carbohydrates:** 0.5g
- **Fiber:** 0g
- **Net Carbs:** 0.5g

These keto marshmallows are a light, guilt-free treat that's perfect for low-carb and keto lifestyles. Enjoy them in hot chocolate, toasted, or as a sweet snack!

Keto Holiday Gummy Bears

These chewy, spiced gummy bears are a fun, low-carb treat with flavors of cinnamon, clove, and a hint of holiday warmth. Perfect for snacking or adding to a holiday dessert tray!

Ingredients:

- 1 cup water
- 2 tablespoons unflavored gelatin powder
- 2–3 tablespoons powdered erythritol (or preferred keto-friendly sweetener)
- 1/2 teaspoon cinnamon
- 1/4 teaspoon ground cloves
- 1/4 teaspoon ground ginger (optional, for extra warmth)
- 1/2 teaspoon vanilla extract
- 1/4 teaspoon liquid stevia or monk fruit sweetener (optional, for added sweetness)

Instructions:

1. **Prepare the Gelatin Mixture:**
   - In a small saucepan, add the water and sprinkle the gelatin powder over the top. Let it sit for 5 minutes to allow the gelatin to bloom.
2. **Add Sweetener and Spices:**
   - Place the saucepan over low heat and add the powdered erythritol, cinnamon, cloves, ginger (if using), and vanilla extract.
   - Stir the mixture constantly until the gelatin and sweetener dissolve completely. Be careful not to let the mixture boil; just heat it enough to dissolve the ingredients.
   - Taste the mixture and add liquid stevia or monk fruit sweetener if additional sweetness is desired.
3. **Pour into Molds:**
   - Using a dropper, fill silicone gummy bear molds with the mixture. (Alternatively, pour the mixture into a shallow baking dish and cut it into small squares once set.)

        ○ Place the molds in the fridge and allow the gummy bears to set for about 1–2 hours, or until firm.
 4. **Remove and Serve:**
        ○ Once set, pop the gummy bears out of the molds. Enjoy immediately, or store them in an airtight container in the fridge for up to one week.

Nutrional Information (per 10 gummy bears, assuming 50 gummy bears total):

- **Calories:** 5
- **Fat:** 0g
- **Protein:** 1g
- **Total Carbohydrates:** 0.5g
- **Fiber:** 0g
- **Net Carbs:** 0.5g

These keto holiday spiced gummy bears are a festive, guilt-free treat with the warm flavors of cinnamon and clove. They're fun to make, low in carbs, and perfect for the holiday season!

White Chocolate Peppermint Bark

This rich, creamy peppermint bark is perfect for the holidays, bringing all the classic flavors of peppermint and white chocolate without the sugar.

Ingredients:

- 1 cup sugar-free white chocolate chips
- 1 tablespoon coconut oil
- 1/2 teaspoon peppermint extract
- Optional: 1–2 sugar-free peppermint candies, crushed (for garnish)

Instructions:

1. **Prepare the White Chocolate Mixture:**
   - In a microwave-safe bowl, combine the sugar-free white chocolate chips and coconut oil.
   - Microwave in 20-second intervals, stirring in between, until fully melted and smooth.
   - Stir in the peppermint extract.
2. **Spread the Bark:**
   - Line a baking sheet with parchment paper. Pour the melted white chocolate mixture onto the parchment and spread it evenly into a thin layer, about 1/4 inch thick.
3. **Add Peppermint Garnish:**
   - Sprinkle the crushed sugar-free peppermint candies over the top of the white chocolate while it's still soft.
4. **Set the Bark:**
   - Place the baking sheet in the fridge for 30 minutes or until the bark is fully set and firm.
5. **Break and Serve:**
   - Once set, break the bark into pieces.
   - Store the bark in an airtight container in the fridge for up to two weeks.

Nutritional Information (per 1 oz piece, assuming 10 pieces)

- **Calories:** 100
- **Fat:** 9g
- **Protein:** 1g
- **Total Carbohydrates:** 4g
- **Fiber:** 2g
- **Net Carbs:** 2g

Enjoy this festive Keto White Chocolate Peppermint Bark as a guilt-free holiday treat! Perfect for sharing, gifting, or indulging while keeping your carbs low.

Classic Chocolate Fudge

This smooth, chocolatey fudge is quick to make and only requires a few ingredients. It's ideal for a holiday treat or an everyday keto dessert.

Ingredients:

- 1/2 cup unsalted butter
- 1/2 cup heavy cream
- 1 cup sugar-free dark chocolate chips (85% cacao or higher)
- 1/4 cup powdered erythritol (or preferred keto-friendly sweetener)
- 1 teaspoon vanilla extract
- 1/4 teaspoon salt

Instructions:

1. **Prepare the Base:**
   - In a small saucepan over medium heat, melt the butter and heavy cream together, stirring frequently.
   - Once the butter has melted, reduce the heat to low and add the sugar-free chocolate chips and powdered erythritol.
2. **Melt and Combine:**
   - Stir constantly until the chocolate chips have fully melted and the mixture is smooth and glossy. Be careful not to let it boil.
3. **Add Flavoring:**
   - Remove from heat and stir in the vanilla extract and salt, mixing until well incorporated.
4. **Pour and Set:**
   - Line a small 8x4-inch loaf pan with parchment paper, leaving some overhang for easy removal. Pour the fudge mixture into the pan, spreading it into an even layer.
   - Refrigerate for at least 2 hours, or until fully set.

5. **Cut and Serve:**
    - Once set, lift the fudge out of the pan using the parchment paper and cut it into squares.
6. **Store:**
    - Store the fudge in an airtight container in the fridge for up to two weeks.

Nutritional Information (per piece, assuming 16 pieces):

- **Calories:** 100
- **Fat:** 10g
- **Protein:** 1g
- **Total Carbohydrates:** 3g
- **Fiber:** 1g
- **Net Carbs:** 2g

This keto chocolate fudge is a rich, creamy treat that's perfect for any chocolate lover following a low-carb lifestyle. Enjoy it as a guilt-free dessert!

Cranberry Pistachio Bark

This cranberry pistachio bark is a beautiful, festive dessert that combines creamy sugar-free white chocolate, crunchy pistachios, and tart cranberries—all without the carbs!

Ingredients:

- 1 cup sugar-free white chocolate chips
- 1 tablespoon coconut oil
- 1/4 cup unsweetened dried cranberries (look for low-carb, unsweetened varieties or make your own by dehydrating fresh cranberries without added sugar)
- 1/4 cup shelled pistachios, roughly chopped

Instructions:

1. **Prepare the White Chocolate Mixture:**
   - In a microwave-safe bowl, combine the sugar-free white chocolate chips and coconut oil.
   - Microwave in 20-second intervals, stirring in between, until fully melted and smooth.
2. **Add Toppings:**
   - Stir half of the chopped pistachios and unsweetened dried cranberries into the melted chocolate mixture.
3. **Spread the Bark:**
   - Line a baking sheet with parchment paper. Pour the chocolate mixture onto the parchment paper and spread it into an even layer, about 1/4 inch thick.
4. **Sprinkle Remaining Toppings:**
   - Sprinkle the remaining chopped pistachios and cranberries evenly over the top of the melted chocolate, pressing them lightly to set into the chocolate.
5. **Set the Bark:**
   - Place the baking sheet in the fridge for 30 minutes or until the bark is fully set and firm.
6. **Break and Serve:**
   - Once set, break the bark into pieces.

- Store the bark in an airtight container in the fridge for up to two weeks.

Nutritional Information (per piece, assuming 10 pieces)

- **Calories:** 90
- **Fat:** 8g
- **Protein:** 1g
- **Total Carbohydrates:** 4g
- **Fiber:** 2g
- **Net Carbs:** 2g

This keto Cranberry Pistachio Bark is a delicious and festive way to enjoy the flavors of the season while staying low-carb. It's perfect for gifting or as a holiday treat!

Peanut Butter Fudge

This peanut butter fudge is quick to make with a few simple ingredients. It's rich, creamy, and has a delightful peanut butter flavor that makes it hard to resist!

Ingredients:

- 1/2 cup unsalted butter
- 1 cup natural creamy peanut butter (no added sugar)
- 1/2 cup powdered erythritol (or your preferred keto-friendly sweetener)
- 1 teaspoon vanilla extract
- 1/4 teaspoon salt

Instructions:

1. **Melt the Butter and Peanut Butter:**
   - In a medium saucepan over low heat, melt the butter. Add the peanut butter and stir until the mixture is smooth and fully combined.
2. **Sweeten and Flavor:**
   - Add the powdered erythritol, vanilla extract, and salt. Stir well until all ingredients are fully incorporated and the mixture is smooth.
3. **Pour and Set:**
   - Line an 8x4-inch loaf pan with parchment paper, leaving some overhang for easy removal.
   - Pour the fudge mixture into the pan, spreading it out evenly with a spatula.
4. **Chill:**
   - Place the fudge in the fridge for at least 2 hours, or until it's fully set.
5. **Cut and Serve:**
   - Once set, lift the fudge out of the pan using the parchment paper and cut it into squares.
6. **Store:**
   - Store the fudge in an airtight container in the fridge for up to two weeks.

Nutritional Information (per piece, assuming 16 pieces)

- **Calories:** 110
- **Fat:** 10g
- **Protein:** 2g
- **Total Carbohydrates:** 3g
- **Fiber:** 1g
- **Net Carbs:** 2g

This keto peanut butter fudge is creamy, rich, and low in carbs, making it a satisfying treat to enjoy while staying on track with your keto lifestyle!

Layered Peppermint Fudge

This layered peppermint fudge features a chocolate layer topped with a creamy peppermint layer, giving it a festive look and delicious flavor without the carbs.

Ingredients:

For the Chocolate Layer:

- 1/2 cup unsalted butter
- 1/2 cup heavy cream
- 1 cup sugar-free dark chocolate chips (85% cacao or higher)
- 1/4 cup powdered erythritol (or preferred keto sweetener)
- 1/2 teaspoon vanilla extract

For the Peppermint Layer:

- 1/2 cup coconut butter (or additional unsalted butter, if coconut butter is unavailable)
- 1/4 cup powdered erythritol
- 1/2 teaspoon peppermint extract
- Optional: a few drops of red food coloring for a holiday swirl effect
- Optional: crushed sugar-free peppermint candies for garnish

Instructions:

1. **Make the Chocolate Layer:**
    - In a small saucepan over low heat, melt the butter and heavy cream together, stirring frequently.
    - Add the sugar-free chocolate chips and powdered erythritol, stirring until smooth and fully melted.
    - Remove from heat and stir in the vanilla extract.
    - Pour the chocolate mixture into an 8x4-inch loaf pan lined with parchment paper, spreading it evenly.
    - Place the pan in the fridge for about 30 minutes, or until the chocolate layer is set.

2. **Make the Peppermint Layer:**
   - In a separate saucepan, melt the coconut butter (or additional unsalted butter) over low heat.
   - Stir in the powdered erythritol and peppermint extract until fully combined.
   - Optional: Add a few drops of red food coloring, swirling lightly to create a festive holiday look.
   - Pour the peppermint mixture over the chilled chocolate layer, spreading it evenly.
3. **Add Garnish and Chill:**
   - If desired, sprinkle crushed sugar-free peppermint candies over the peppermint layer for a festive touch.
   - Return the pan to the fridge for at least 1 hour, or until fully set.
4. **Cut and Serve:**
   - Once set, lift the fudge out of the pan using the parchment paper and cut it into squares.
5. **Store:**
   - Store the fudge in an airtight container in the fridge for up to two weeks.

Nutritional Information (per piece, assuming 16 pieces)

- **Calories:** 120
- **Fat:** 11g
- **Protein:** 1g
- **Total Carbohydrates:** 4g
- **Fiber:** 2g
- **Net Carbs:** 2g

Salted Keto Caramels

These salted caramels are smooth and chewy, with the perfect balance of sweetness and salt. They make a great low-carb treat or holiday gift.

Ingredients:

- 1/2 cup unsalted butter
- 1/2 cup heavy cream
- 1/3 cup powdered erythritol (or your preferred keto sweetener)
- 1 teaspoon vanilla extract
- 1/4 teaspoon salt
- Flaky sea salt, for sprinkling

Instructions:

1. **Prepare the Caramel Base:**
    - In a medium saucepan over medium heat, melt the butter, stirring frequently until it begins to brown slightly (about 5 minutes).
    - Lower the heat to medium-low and add the heavy cream and powdered erythritol. Stir until fully combined.
2. **Cook the Caramel:**
    - Continue to cook the mixture over medium-low heat, stirring constantly to prevent burning, until it thickens and turns a rich caramel color. This should take about 10–15 minutes.

- o Remove from heat and stir in the vanilla extract and salt.
3. **Pour and Set:**
    - o Line a small 8x4-inch loaf pan with parchment paper, leaving a bit of overhang for easy removal.
    - o Pour the caramel mixture into the prepared pan and spread it into an even layer.
    - o Sprinkle the top with flaky sea salt for a salted caramel flavor.
4. **Chill:**
    - o Place the pan in the fridge and let the caramels set for at least 1 hour, or until firm.
5. **Cut and Serve:**
    - o Once set, lift the caramels out of the pan using the parchment paper and cut them into small squares.
6. **Store:**
    - o Store the caramels in an airtight container in the fridge for up to two weeks.

Nutritional Information (per piece, assuming 16 pieces)

- **Calories:** 70
- **Fat:** 7g
- **Protein:** 0.5g
- **Total Carbohydrates:** 1g
- **Fiber:** 0g
- **Net Carbs:** 1g

These salted keto caramels are a delightful, chewy treat that's perfect for keto snacking or holiday gifting. Enjoy the sweetness without the carbs!

Holiday Taffy

This sugar-free taffy is soft, chewy, and comes in festive flavors like peppermint and cinnamon. It's a fun, low-carb treat to enjoy or give as a holiday gift.

Ingredients

- 1/2 cup unsalted butter
- 1/2 cup heavy cream
- 1/3 cup powdered erythritol (or preferred keto-friendly sweetener)
- 1/4 teaspoon salt
- 1/2 teaspoon peppermint extract (or cinnamon extract, or any holiday flavor)
- Optional: a few drops of red or green food coloring (for festive flair)

Instructions:

1. **Prepare the Base:**
    - In a medium saucepan over medium heat, melt the butter and heavy cream together, stirring constantly.
2. **Sweeten and Flavor:**
    - Add the powdered erythritol and salt, continuing to stir until fully combined. Bring the mixture to a gentle simmer, stirring continuously.
3. **Cook the Taffy:**
    - Reduce the heat to low and continue to cook, stirring constantly, until the mixture thickens and turns a light golden color. This should take around 10–15 minutes.
    - Once the mixture reaches a chewy consistency, remove it from heat and quickly stir in the peppermint or cinnamon extract and a few drops of food coloring if using.
4. **Cool and Stretch:**
    - Allow the mixture to cool slightly until it's safe to handle. Grease your hands with a little butter or coconut oil, then stretch and pull the taffy for about 5

minutes to incorporate air. This will give it a light, chewy texture.
    - Shape the taffy into small logs or twist into pieces.
5. **Set and Serve:**
    - Place the taffy pieces on parchment paper and allow them to cool completely.
    - Wrap each piece in wax paper or parchment paper to prevent sticking.
6. **Store:**
    - Store the taffy in an airtight container at room temperature or in the fridge for up to one week.

Nutritional Information (per piece, assuming 20 pieces)

- **Calories:** 35
- **Fat:** 4g
- **Protein:** 0g
- **Total Carbohydrates:** 1g
- **Fiber:** 0g
- **Net Carbs:** 1g

This keto holiday taffy is a festive, chewy treat with your favorite seasonal flavors. Enjoy it without the carbs or sugar spikes!

Gingerbread Caramel Chews

These caramels are creamy, chewy, and spiced with gingerbread flavors like ginger, cinnamon, and nutmeg. Perfect for holiday snacking or gifting!

Ingredients:

- 1/2 cup unsalted butter
- 1/2 cup heavy cream
- 1/3 cup powdered erythritol (or preferred keto-friendly sweetener)
- 1/2 teaspoon ground ginger
- 1/2 teaspoon ground cinnamon
- 1/4 teaspoon ground nutmeg
- 1/8 teaspoon ground cloves
- 1 teaspoon vanilla extract
- 1/4 teaspoon salt

Instructions:

1. **Prepare the Caramel Base:**
   - In a medium saucepan over medium heat, melt the butter. Add the heavy cream and powdered erythritol, stirring to combine.
2. **Add the Spices:**
   - Stir in the ground ginger, cinnamon, nutmeg, and cloves. Keep stirring until the spices are well distributed in the caramel mixture.
3. **Cook the Caramel:**
   - Continue cooking the mixture over medium-low heat, stirring constantly, until it thickens and turns a rich caramel color (about 10–15 minutes). The mixture should be smooth and start to pull away slightly from the sides of the saucepan.
   - Remove the saucepan from heat and stir in the vanilla extract and salt.
4. **Pour and Set:**
   - Line an 8x4-inch loaf pan with parchment paper, leaving some overhang for easy removal. Pour the

caramel mixture into the prepared pan, spreading it into an even layer.
5. **Cool and Cut:**
    - Allow the caramel to cool at room temperature for about an hour, then transfer it to the fridge to set completely, about 1–2 hours.
    - Once set, lift the caramel out of the pan using the parchment paper and cut it into small squares.
6. **Store:**
    - Wrap each caramel individually in wax paper or parchment paper. Store in an airtight container in the fridge for up to two weeks.

Nutritional Information (per piece, assuming 16 pieces)

- **Calories:** 60
- **Fat:** 6g
- **Protein:** 0.5g
- **Total Carbohydrates:** 1.5g
- **Fiber:** 0g
- **Net Carbs:** 1.5g

These Keto Gingerbread Caramel Chews offer a delightful blend of spices with a chewy, caramel texture that's perfect for the holidays. Enjoy them as a low-carb treat to celebrate the season!

Coconut Macadamia Caramels

These buttery, chewy caramels are infused with coconut flavor and studded with macadamia nuts, making them a deliciously decadent treat!

Ingredients:

- 1/2 cup unsalted butter
- 1/4 cup heavy cream
- 1/4 cup canned coconut cream (thick, unsweetened)
- 1/3 cup powdered erythritol (or your preferred keto-friendly sweetener)
- 1/4 teaspoon salt
- 1 teaspoon vanilla extract
- 1/4 teaspoon coconut extract (optional, for extra coconut flavor)
- 1/2 cup macadamia nuts, chopped

Instructions:

1. **Prepare the Caramel Base:**
   - In a medium saucepan over medium heat, melt the butter. Add the heavy cream, coconut cream, and powdered erythritol, stirring until smooth.
2. **Cook the Caramel:**
   - Continue to cook the mixture over medium-low heat, stirring constantly to avoid burning, until it thickens and turns a golden caramel color, about 10–15 minutes.
   - Remove the saucepan from heat and stir in the salt, vanilla extract, and coconut extract, if using.
3. **Add the Macadamias:**
   - Stir the chopped macadamia nuts into the caramel mixture until evenly distributed.
4. **Pour and Set:**
   - Line an 8x4-inch loaf pan with parchment paper, leaving an overhang for easy removal. Pour the

caramel mixture into the prepared pan and spread it into an even layer.

5. **Cool and Cut:**
    - Let the caramel cool at room temperature for about 1 hour, then transfer it to the fridge to set completely, about 1–2 hours.
    - Once set, lift the caramel out of the pan using the parchment paper and cut it into small squares.
6. **Store:**
    - Store the caramels in an airtight container in the fridge for up to two weeks.

Nutritional Information (per piece, assuming 16 pieces):

- **Calories:** 80
- **Fat:** 8g
- **Protein:** 0.5g
- **Total Carbohydrates:** 2g
- **Fiber:** 0.5g
- **Net Carbs:** 1.5g

These Keto Coconut Macadamia Caramels are creamy, nutty, and perfectly chewy with a hint of coconut flavor. They're a delicious low-carb treat to satisfy your sweet cravings!

Hot Cocoa Fat Bombs

These creamy, chocolatey fat bombs have a smooth texture with a touch of marshmallow flavor. They're easy to make and a delicious way to enjoy a hot cocoa-inspired treat while staying low-carb.

Ingredients:

- 1/2 cup unsalted butter, softened
- 1/4 cup coconut oil, softened
- 1/4 cup heavy cream
- 1/3 cup unsweetened cocoa powder
- 1/4 cup powdered erythritol (or your preferred keto-friendly sweetener)
- 1/2 teaspoon vanilla extract
- 1/4 teaspoon marshmallow extract (optional, for marshmallow flavor)

Instructions:

1. **Prepare the Base:**
    - In a mixing bowl, beat the softened butter and coconut oil together until smooth and creamy.
2. **Add Cocoa and Sweetener:**
    - Add the heavy cream, unsweetened cocoa powder, and powdered erythritol. Mix until well combined and smooth.
3. **Flavoring:**
    - Stir in the vanilla extract and marshmallow extract, if using. Taste the mixture and adjust sweetness or flavoring to preference.
4. **Shape the Fat Bombs:**
    - Line a mini muffin pan with liners or use silicone molds. Scoop the mixture into each mold, smoothing the tops.
5. **Set the Fat Bombs:**
    - Place the pan in the freezer for about 30 minutes or until the fat bombs are firm.

6. **Serve and Store:**
    - Once set, remove the fat bombs from the molds. Store them in an airtight container in the fridge for up to two weeks or in the freezer for longer storage.

Nutritional Information (per fat bomb, assuming 12 fat bombs):

- **Calories:** 90
- **Fat:** 9g
- **Protein:** 0.5g
- **Total Carbohydrates:** 2g
- **Fiber:** 1g
- **Net Carbs:** 1g

These Keto Hot Cocoa Fat Bombs are a creamy, chocolatey treat with just a hint of marshmallow flavor. They're perfect for a quick snack or dessert on a keto diet! Enjoy!

Eggnog Fat Bombs

These rich, creamy fat bombs are infused with classic eggnog spices like nutmeg and cinnamon. They're a delicious and satisfying holiday snack that fits into a low-carb lifestyle.

Ingredients:

- 1/2 cup unsalted butter, softened
- 1/4 cup coconut oil, softened
- 1/4 cup cream cheese, softened
- 1/4 cup heavy cream
- 1/4 cup powdered erythritol (or preferred keto-friendly sweetener)
- 1/2 teaspoon vanilla extract
- 1/2 teaspoon rum extract (optional, for eggnog flavor)
- 1/4 teaspoon ground nutmeg
- 1/4 teaspoon ground cinnamon
- Optional: pinch of ground cloves (for extra holiday flavor)

Instructions:

1. **Prepare the Base:**
    - In a mixing bowl, beat together the softened butter, coconut oil, and cream cheese until smooth and creamy.
2. **Add the Cream and Sweetener:**
    - Add the heavy cream and powdered erythritol. Continue to mix until fully incorporated and smooth.
3. **Flavoring and Spices:**
    - Stir in the vanilla extract, rum extract (if using), ground nutmeg, cinnamon, and cloves (if using). Mix well to ensure the spices are evenly distributed.
4. **Shape the Fat Bombs:**
    - Line a mini muffin pan with liners or use silicone molds. Scoop the mixture into each mold, smoothing the tops.
5. **Set the Fat Bombs:**
    - Place the pan in the freezer for about 30 minutes or until the fat bombs are firm.

6. **Serve and Store:**
   - Once set, remove the fat bombs from the molds. Store them in an airtight container in the fridge for up to two weeks or in the freezer for longer storage.

Nutritional Information (per fat bomb, assuming 12 fat bombs)

- **Calories:** 90
- **Fat:** 9g
- **Protein:** 0.5g
- **Total Carbohydrates:** 1.5g
- **Fiber:** 0g
- **Net Carbs:** 1.5g

These Keto Eggnog Fat Bombs are a perfect way to enjoy the creamy, spiced flavors of eggnog while keeping it low-carb and keto-friendly. Enjoy the holiday season with these delightful bites!

Peppermint Mocha Fat Bombs

These fat bombs combine rich cocoa, coffee, and refreshing peppermint for a delicious keto-friendly treat with minimal carbs.

Ingredients:

- 1/2 cup unsalted butter, softened
- 1/4 cup coconut oil, softened
- 1/4 cup cream cheese, softened
- 1/4 cup heavy cream
- 1 tablespoon instant coffee powder (or 1 teaspoon espresso powder)
- 1/4 cup powdered erythritol (or preferred keto-friendly sweetener)
- 2 tablespoons unsweetened cocoa powder
- 1/2 teaspoon peppermint extract

Instructions:

1. **Prepare the Base:**
   - In a mixing bowl, beat the softened butter, coconut oil, and cream cheese until smooth and creamy.
2. **Add the Flavoring:**
   - In a small bowl, dissolve the instant coffee powder in the heavy cream, then add it to the butter mixture. Stir well to incorporate.
   - Add the powdered erythritol, unsweetened cocoa powder, and peppermint extract. Mix until all ingredients are fully combined and smooth.
3. **Shape the Fat Bombs:**
   - Line a mini muffin pan with liners or use silicone molds. Scoop the mixture into each mold, smoothing the tops.
4. **Set the Fat Bombs:**
   - Place the pan in the freezer for about 30 minutes or until the fat bombs are firm.

5. **Serve and Store:**
    - Once set, remove the fat bombs from the molds. Store them in an airtight container in the fridge for up to two weeks or in the freezer for longer storage.

Nutritional Information (per fat bomb, assuming 12 fat bombs)

- **Calories:** 90
- **Fat:** 9g
- **Protein:** 0.5g
- **Total Carbohydrates:** 2g
- **Fiber:** 1g
- **Net Carbs:** 1g

These Keto Peppermint Mocha Fat Bombs bring the warm flavors of peppermint and coffee together in a creamy, low-carb treat. Perfect for a quick, cozy snack anytime!

Cinnamon Roll Fat Bombs

These creamy, cinnamon-spiced fat bombs are sweet, buttery, and packed with flavor. They're an easy, low-carb treat to satisfy your cravings for something cozy!

Ingredients:

For the Fat Bombs:

- 1/2 cup unsalted butter, softened
- 1/4 cup coconut oil, softened
- 1/4 cup cream cheese, softened
- 1/4 cup powdered erythritol (or preferred keto-friendly sweetener)
- 1 teaspoon vanilla extract
- 1 teaspoon ground cinnamon

For the Cinnamon Swirl Topping:

- 1 tablespoon melted butter
- 1/2 teaspoon ground cinnamon
- 1 tablespoon powdered erythritol (or preferred keto sweetener)

Instructions:

1. **Prepare the Base:**
   - In a mixing bowl, beat the softened butter, coconut oil, and cream cheese until smooth and creamy.
   - Add the powdered erythritol, vanilla extract, and ground cinnamon. Mix until fully incorporated and smooth.
2. **Shape the Fat Bombs:**
   - Line a mini muffin pan with liners or use silicone molds. Scoop the mixture into each mold, smoothing the tops.

3. **Add the Cinnamon Swirl Topping:**
   - In a small bowl, mix together the melted butter, cinnamon, and powdered erythritol to create the swirl topping.
   - Drizzle a small amount of the cinnamon mixture over each fat bomb and swirl it with a toothpick to create a cinnamon roll effect.
4. **Set the Fat Bombs:**
   - Place the pan in the freezer for about 30 minutes, or until the fat bombs are firm.
5. **Serve and Store:**
   - Once set, remove the fat bombs from the molds. Store them in an airtight container in the fridge for up to two weeks or in the freezer for longer storage.

Nutritional Information (per fat bomb, assuming 12 fat bombs)

- **Calories:** 95
- **Fat:** 10g
- **Protein:** 0.5g
- **Total Carbohydrates:** 2g
- **Fiber:** 0.5g
- **Net Carbs:** 1.5g

These Keto Cinnamon Roll Fat Bombs are the perfect cozy, low-carb treat for winter! Enjoy the warm, spiced flavor without the carbs.

Sugar Free Sweeteners

When it comes to enjoying sweet treats on a keto lifestyle, choosing the right sugar substitute is key. Not all sweeteners are created equal—each has unique properties, flavors, and impacts on your body. In this chapter, we'll cover some of the most popular sugar-free sweeteners used in keto cooking and baking, including how to choose the best one for your recipe.

Why Choose Sugar-Free Sweetners?

Traditional sugar causes blood sugar spikes and takes you out of ketosis, so it's best avoided on a keto diet. Sugar-free sweeteners, however, allow you to add sweetness without the carbs. These alternatives are designed to mimic the flavor and sweetness of sugar without the high glycemic impact. Let's explore some of the most popular options.

Erythritol: The Sugar Alcohol Standard

What It Is: Erythritol is a sugar alcohol naturally found in some fruits. It's one of the most popular sweeteners for keto because it has zero net carbs and a glycemic index of zero.

Best Uses: Erythritol is great for baking because it adds bulk, similar to sugar. It's ideal in cookies, cakes, and even frostings. It crystallizes when cooled, so it's best paired with another sweetener in recipes like custards or caramels to avoid a gritty texture.

Sweetness Level: Erythritol is about 70% as sweet as sugar. In recipes, you may need to use a bit more erythritol than sugar to achieve the desired sweetness.

Pros and Cons:

- **Pros**: Zero net carbs, good for baking, doesn't cause blood sugar spikes.
- **Cons**: Can cause a cooling effect in the mouth, crystallizes in some recipes, and may cause digestive issues for some people.

Quick Tip: Powdered erythritol is easier to dissolve than granulated, making it better for frostings, glazes, or anything that needs a smoother texture.

Stevia: The Natural, Calorie-Free Sweetener

What It Is: Stevia is a plant-derived sweetener that's been used for centuries. It's very sweet, so a little goes a long way. Stevia can be found in liquid drops, powder, or granulated blends.

Best Uses: Stevia works well in beverages, smoothies, and desserts where you need a touch of sweetness. Since it's so sweet, it's not the best for recipes where sugar adds structure, like cookies.

Sweetness Level: Stevia is around 200–300 times sweeter than sugar, so you only need a small amount.

Pros and Cons:

- **Pros**: Zero calories, zero carbs, no impact on blood sugar.
- **Cons**: Some people find it has a bitter aftertaste; it can be tricky to measure and balance in recipes.

Quick Tip: Stevia blends are often mixed with erythritol to balance sweetness and make it easier to measure. Look for these blends if you need to avoid aftertaste and want a more sugar-like experience.

Allulose: The Sugar Substitute That Acts Like Sugar

What It Is: Allulose is a "rare sugar" that's naturally found in figs, raisins, and other fruits. It has the same texture and caramelization ability as sugar but is low in calories and doesn't raise blood glucose levels.

Best Uses: Allulose is excellent in recipes where you need a smooth texture, like caramel, ice cream, or sauces. It dissolves well and won't crystallize like erythritol, making it ideal for fudges and syrups.

Sweetness Level: Allulose is about 70% as sweet as sugar, so you may need slightly more to reach your desired sweetness.

Pros and Cons:

- **Pros**: No crystallization, low-carb, no aftertaste, ideal for caramelizing.
- **Cons**: Slightly more expensive, some people may experience digestive discomfort at high doses.

Quick Tip: If you're making candy or caramel, allulose is your best choice. It browns beautifully and won't recrystallize, giving your sweets the smooth texture you want.

Monk Fruit: The Sweetness of Longevity

What It Is: Monk fruit is a small green melon that's native to southern China. It's named after the Buddhist monks who cultivated it. Monk fruit sweetener is a natural, zero-calorie sweetener extracted from the fruit.

Best Uses: Monk fruit is versatile and can be used in most recipes where you would use erythritol or stevia. It's available in powdered, granulated, and liquid forms, and it's often combined with other sweeteners to balance the sweetness.

Sweetness Level: Monk fruit is 150–200 times sweeter than sugar, so a little goes a long way.

Pros and Cons:

- **Pros**: Zero carbs, doesn't raise blood sugar, no aftertaste when blended properly.
- **Cons**: On its own, it's intensely sweet; usually, it's mixed with other sweeteners, which can impact the flavor and texture of recipes.

Quick Tip: Look for monk fruit-erythritol blends to get a balanced sweetness without any bitterness.

Xylitol: Sweet, But with Caution

What It Is: Xylitol is a sugar alcohol found naturally in some fruits and vegetables. It's low-carb, has a low glycemic index, and tastes very similar to sugar. However, it's important to note that xylitol is highly toxic to dogs, so keep it safely out of reach if you have pets.

Best Uses: Xylitol is excellent for baking, especially in recipes like cookies and muffins where a close match to sugar's texture is needed. It doesn't have the cooling effect of erythritol and behaves more like traditional sugar.

Sweetness Level: Xylitol is about as sweet as sugar, making it easy to substitute in recipes.

Pros and Cons:

- **Pros**: Low glycemic impact, close in taste and texture to sugar, no cooling effect.
- **Cons**: Toxic to dogs, can cause digestive discomfort for some people.

Quick Tip: If you're baking for family without pets, xylitol can be a great choice. But if you have pets, you may want to use an alternative to avoid any risks.

Tips for Choosing the Right Sweetener

1. **For Baking**: Erythritol or xylitol are ideal for baked goods that need structure and bulk. Look for blends with erythritol and stevia for a balanced sweetness.
2. **For Candies and Caramels**: Allulose works best for candies and sauces because it doesn't crystallize.
3. **For Drinks and Frostings**: Stevia, monk fruit, or erythritol powder are great for beverages and frostings where a fine texture is needed.
4. **For Smooth Textures**: Use allulose or powdered erythritol for recipes like fudge, sauces, or syrups to avoid a gritty feel.

Sweetener Conversion Guide

When substituting for sugar in recipes, keep in mind the sweetness levels:

- **Erythritol**: 1.25 times the amount of sugar for equal sweetness
- **Stevia**: About 1/4 teaspoon per cup of sugar (adjust to taste)
- **Allulose**: 1.25 times the amount of sugar for equal sweetness
- **Monk Fruit**: Typically blended with other sweeteners, check package instructions

Final Thoughts

Each of these sweeteners has unique qualities, and experimenting with them can help you find the best fit for your keto lifestyle. With these sugar-free options, you can enjoy all the flavors of sweetness without the carbs. Choose the right sweetener, and you'll be able to indulge in delicious keto treats that make every day feel like a celebration!

Keto Candy Making Tips

Making keto-friendly candy requires a bit of finesse and knowledge of specific techniques to achieve the desired texture, flavor, and appearance without traditional sugar. In this chapter, we'll explore the best practices for creating delicious keto candies that are as satisfying as the real thing. From handling sugar-free sweeteners to mastering textures, here are the top tips for keto candy-making success!

Choosing The Right Sweetener

The sweetener you choose is crucial in keto candy-making, as each type behaves differently. Here are some quick pointers:

- **Allulose** is ideal for candies like caramels, brittles, and fudges because it doesn't crystallize and creates a smooth, chewy texture.
- **Erythritol** works well in hard candies and chocolates, but it can sometimes crystallize, leaving a gritty texture. Powdered erythritol blends can minimize this effect.
- **Monk Fruit-Erythritol Blends** are great for a balanced sweetness and work well in chocolates and fudge. Avoid using them in recipes that require high heat, as they may crystallize.
- **Xylitol** offers a similar sweetness and texture to sugar and doesn't have a cooling effect like erythritol. However, remember to avoid this sweetener if you have pets, as it's highly toxic to dogs.

Creating Smooth Textures

A smooth, creamy texture is essential in keto caramels, fudges, and other soft candies. Here's how to achieve it:

- **Use Powdered Sweeteners**: Granulated sweeteners can create a gritty texture in candies. Powdered versions of erythritol, monk fruit blends, and allulose dissolve more easily and give a smoother result.

- **Keep the Temperature Low and Stir Constantly**: Heating too quickly can lead to uneven textures and crystallization. Cook your candy mixtures over low to medium heat and stir constantly to prevent sticking and ensure a creamy consistency.
- **Add a Fat Component**: Butter, coconut oil, or heavy cream helps create a rich, smooth texture, especially in fudges, toffees, and caramels. These fats contribute to the creamy mouthfeel associated with traditional candies.

Controlling Crystallization

Crystallization can lead to a gritty texture in candy, especially with sugar alcohols like erythritol. Here are a few tips to prevent crystallization:

- **Use Allulose for Smooth Candies**: Allulose doesn't crystallize as it cools, so it's a great choice for soft caramels and fudges.
- **Add a Dash of Salt or Cream of Tartar**: These ingredients help inhibit crystallization, leading to a smoother, creamier texture.
- **Avoid Disturbing the Mixture While It Cools**: Once you've poured your mixture into the mold, let it set without stirring or moving. Disruption can encourage sugar alcohols to crystallize and leave a grainy texture.

Achieving the Perfect Chewy Texture

Chewiness is key in candies like caramels and taffies. Here's how to make your keto candies satisfyingly chewy:

- **Use Heavy Cream or Coconut Cream**: Cream gives a caramel-like chewiness. Avoid milk, as it's lower in fat and may not achieve the desired texture.

- **Heat to the Right Temperature**: Use a candy thermometer and cook the mixture until it reaches the right stage (usually between 245°F and 250°F for chewy caramels).
- **Add Gelatin**: For some keto taffies and gummy candies, adding a small amount of unflavored gelatin can help achieve a chewier, bouncier texture without the carbs.

Workign with Chocolate

Chocolate is a keto candy staple, but sugar-free chocolate can be finicky to work with. Here's how to master keto chocolate treats:

- **Melt Slowly**: Melt sugar-free chocolate over a double boiler or in the microwave in short intervals, stirring frequently to prevent burning.
- **Use Coconut Oil for a Smoother Finish**: Adding a small amount of coconut oil (1 tablespoon per cup of chocolate) helps create a smoother texture and makes the chocolate easier to coat over nuts, truffles, and bars.
- **Tempering Chocolate**: Tempering chocolate helps it set with a glossy finish and a crisp snap. Heat your chocolate to 115°F, then cool it to about 85°F before reheating slightly to 88°F–90°F. This process is optional but useful for professional-looking candies.

Flavoring Keto Candies

Adding flavor to keto candies can take them to the next level. Here's how to infuse flavors without adding carbs:

- **Use Extracts and Oils**: Pure extracts like vanilla, peppermint, almond, and coconut work beautifully in keto candy and add flavor without sugar. A few drops of food-grade essential oils (like peppermint or orange) can also give a potent flavor boost.
- **Spices for Depth**: Spices like cinnamon, ginger, and nutmeg bring a warm, cozy flavor to holiday candies. Use sparingly to avoid overpowering the candy.

- **Acid Balance**: For fruity candies, a few drops of lemon or lime juice can enhance flavor and cut through sweetness. Acid can also prevent crystallization in some recipes.

Perfecting Appearance and Presentation

The look of keto candies is part of the experience. Here's how to get professional-looking results:

- **Molds for Shape**: Silicone molds are perfect for fat bombs, fudge, and gummy candies. They're easy to use, and the candy pops out cleanly without sticking.
- **Sprinkle Finishing Touches**: Add crushed nuts, shredded coconut, sea salt, or a dusting of cocoa powder for visual appeal and added texture.
- **Use a Sharp Knife**: For neat, clean edges on caramels and fudge, chill the candy first, then cut with a sharp knife.

Storage and Serving Keto Candy

Proper storage can help maintain the texture and flavor of your keto candies:

- **Refrigerate for Freshness**: Many keto candies, especially those with cream, butter, or coconut oil, need to be stored in the fridge to maintain their texture and freshness.
- **Serve at Room Temperature**: Allow candies to come to room temperature before serving for the best texture and flavor, especially for caramels and fudge.
- **Freeze for Long-Term Storage**: Keto candies can often be frozen for up to three months. Just be sure to wrap them tightly to prevent freezer burn.

Final Thoughts

With these tips, you're ready to take your keto candy-making skills to the next level. Creating sugar-free, low-carb treats may seem challenging at first, but with the right techniques, you can craft candies that are every bit as delicious as their traditional counterparts. Whether you're making chewy caramels, creamy fudge, or rich chocolate truffles, these tips will help you achieve the perfect texture, flavor, and appearance.

Dive in, experiment, and enjoy the sweet rewards of keto candy-making! With a little practice, you'll be able to satisfy your sweet tooth without compromising your keto goals.

Storage & Shelf Life of Keto Candies

When you've put time and effort into making delicious keto candies, storing them correctly ensures they stay fresh, flavorful, and safe to eat. Because keto candies often rely on ingredients like butter, cream, and sugar-free sweeteners, they can have different storage requirements from traditional sugary treats. In this chapter, we'll cover storage guidelines for various types of keto candies, tips to extend freshness, and recommendations for long-term storage.

General Storage Tips for Keto Candies

Most keto candies require careful storage to maintain their texture, flavor, and quality. Here are a few general tips to get you started:

- **Use Airtight Containers**: Store your candies in an airtight container to prevent exposure to moisture and air, which can cause texture changes and spoilage.
- **Separate Layers with Parchment Paper**: If your candies are sticky or have coatings that may rub off, use parchment paper to layer them. This is especially helpful for fudge, truffles, or candies with chocolate coatings.
- **Avoid Direct Sunlight and Heat**: Heat can melt or damage the texture of keto candies, particularly those made with chocolate, butter, or coconut oil. Keep them in a cool, dark place.

Refrigerating Keto Candies

Many keto candies benefit from being stored in the refrigerator, especially those containing dairy products like cream or butter. Here's a quick guide to the types of candies that should be refrigerated:

- **Candies with Dairy**: Fudge, caramels, and fat bombs with ingredients like heavy cream, cream cheese, or butter need to be refrigerated to prevent spoilage. These candies will generally last up to two weeks in the fridge.
- **Chocolate-Based Candies**: Chocolate fat bombs, truffles, and bark can also be stored in the fridge to keep them from melting. Chocolate candies tend to stay fresh in the fridge for about two to three weeks.
- **Nut-Based Candies**: Nut brittles, pralines, or nut clusters can be stored at room temperature if you'll consume them within a week. Otherwise, refrigerating them can help keep the nuts fresh and crunchy.

Best Practice: Place refrigerated candies on the counter for 10–15 minutes before serving to let them come to room temperature. This helps them soften slightly for a better mouthfeel.

Freezing Keto Candies for Long-Term Storage

Freezing keto candies is an excellent way to extend their shelf life without compromising flavor or texture. Follow these tips to freeze your homemade candies successfully:

- **Wrap Individually**: For fudge, caramels, or fat bombs, wrap each piece individually in plastic wrap or parchment paper before placing them in a freezer-safe container or resealable bag. This keeps them from sticking together and makes it easy to take out individual portions.
- **Use Freezer-Safe Containers**: Choose containers that are specifically made for freezing to prevent freezer burn and protect the candies from moisture. Resealable freezer bags or silicone containers are ideal options.
- **Label with Date**: Keto candies can last in the freezer for up to three months. Label each container with the date so you can track how long they've been stored.

Quick Tip: Some candies, like truffles and fat bombs, can be enjoyed straight from the freezer for a firmer texture, while others, like fudge or caramel, should be thawed in the fridge overnight before eating.

Storing Specific Types of Keto Candies

Different types of candies have unique storage requirements. Here's a breakdown to help you store each type for maximum freshness:

- **Fudge**: Keto fudge is best stored in the fridge. Wrap it tightly or keep it in an airtight container to prevent it from absorbing other fridge odors. Fudge will last about 2–3 weeks refrigerated and up to 3 months frozen.
- **Caramels**: Keto caramels should be wrapped individually in wax paper and stored in the fridge to prevent them from melting. They'll keep for about 2 weeks in the fridge or up to 3 months in the freezer.
- **Chocolate Barks and Peppermint Bark**: These can be stored at room temperature for about a week in a cool, dark place, away from direct sunlight. For longer storage, keep them in the fridge for up to 3 weeks or in the freezer for up to 3 months.
- **Nut Brittle and Toffees**: Nut brittle and toffee are the most stable at room temperature. Keep them in an airtight container at room temperature, and they should last up to 2 weeks. If you need longer storage, place them in the fridge for up to a month.
- **Truffles and Fat Bombs**: These are best stored in the fridge, as they're typically made with ingredients like cream, butter, or coconut oil. They'll stay fresh for about 2 weeks in the fridge or up to 3 months in the freezer.
- **Gummy Candies**: Keto gummy candies made with gelatin can be stored at room temperature if consumed within a few days. Otherwise, refrigerate them for up to 2 weeks to maintain their texture and flavor.

Preventing Common Storage Issues

Keto candies, particularly those made with sugar substitutes, can sometimes present unique storage challenges. Here's how to handle common issues:

- **Crystallization**: Erythritol-based candies may crystallize over time, which can create a gritty texture. Storing these candies in the fridge can help minimize crystallization.
- **Softening and Melting**: Fat bombs and chocolates made with coconut oil can soften or melt at room temperature. Keep these in the fridge, especially in warm climates, to maintain their shape.
- **Absorbing Fridge Odors**: Candies like fudge and caramel can sometimes absorb strong odors from the fridge. Store them in airtight containers or tightly wrap them in plastic wrap to prevent this.
- **Preventing Freezer Burn**: Always store keto candies in freezer-safe containers and avoid leaving them uncovered. Freezer burn can alter texture and flavor, so tightly wrapping each piece and using containers with airtight lids will help.

Serving Tips for Stored Keto Candies

When you're ready to serve stored keto candies, these tips can help you present them at their best:

- **Room Temperature for Optimal Texture**: Candies like fudge, caramels, and fat bombs should be allowed to warm up slightly at room temperature before serving for the best flavor and texture.
- **Slice and Portion Before Storing**: If you're freezing larger pieces of fudge or bark, consider slicing them into serving-size pieces before freezing. This makes it easier to defrost only the amount you need.

- **Avoid Repeated Freezing and Thawing**: Freezing and thawing multiple times can affect texture, so only take out what you plan to use to maintain the quality of the remaining candy.

Final Thoughts

Storing keto candies properly ensures you'll have delicious treats ready to enjoy whenever cravings strike. By following these best practices, you can extend the freshness of your candies and avoid issues like crystallization or spoilage. Whether you're making fudge, brittle, or fat bombs, these storage techniques will keep your treats in perfect condition.

Homemade keto candies deserve the best care, so take the time to store them right. This way, you can savor each bite of your hard work—fresh, flavorful, and perfectly preserved.

Gift Wrapping Ideas

One of the best parts of making keto candies is sharing them with friends and family. Thoughtful, creative packaging can elevate your homemade treats into beautiful, personal gifts. In this chapter, we'll explore various ways to wrap and present your keto candies for gifting, ensuring your creations look as good as they taste!

Choosing the Right Packaging Materials

Before getting started, consider the type of candy you're gifting, as some packaging materials work better for different candies:

- **Moisture-Sensitive Candies** (like fudge or truffles): Opt for airtight containers or jars to maintain texture and freshness.
- **Dry or Hard Candies** (like brittle or toffee): Small bags, boxes, or tins are great options, as they don't need to be airtight.
- **Delicate Candies** (like fat bombs or chocolates): Line packages with parchment paper or use candy liners to prevent them from sticking or breaking.

With this in mind, let's dive into the creative ways to wrap and present your keto candies.

Classic Mason Jars

Mason jars are timeless for candy gifting, adding a rustic, homemade touch. Here's how to make them festive and personal:

- **Layer the Candies**: Fill the jar with layers of different candies for an eye-catching presentation. For example, start with a layer of keto fudge, then add peppermint bark, and top it off with a few fat bombs.
- **Add a Label or Tag**: Use chalkboard labels, kraft paper, or printable tags to write the candy names and any storage instructions. Personalize each jar with a hand-written message or the recipient's name.
- **Decorate the Lid**: Wrap a circle of festive fabric around the lid, secure with a ribbon or twine, and add a sprig of rosemary or pine for a holiday feel.

Best For: Fudge, fat bombs, caramels, or brittle.

Small Tin Boxes

Tins are ideal for candies that need a bit of protection, and they come in a range of sizes, shapes, and designs. Here's how to personalize them:

- **Line with Parchment Paper**: Cut parchment paper to fit the tin's bottom and sides. This adds a touch of elegance and keeps candies from sticking to the tin.
- **Add Dividers for Variety**: If you're including different types of candy, create small dividers with pieces of parchment paper or cardstock to separate each type.
- **Seal with a Decorative Label**: Seal the tin with a festive sticker or label and tie a ribbon around the tin's edge.

Best For: Brittle, toffees, nut clusters, or truffles.

Clear Cellophane Bags

Clear cellophane bags are affordable, versatile, and showcase the candies beautifully. They're perfect for smaller gifts or individual servings:

- **Bundle with a Twist Tie**: Fill each bag with a handful of candy, twist the top, and secure it with a decorative twist tie or small ribbon.
- **Layer for Visual Appeal**: Layer different candies, stacking various colors and textures to create a visually appealing presentation.
- **Add a Tag or Recipe Card**: Attach a tag with the candy's name and ingredients, or include a small recipe card if you're gifting homemade treats to keto enthusiasts.

Best For: Fudge squares, caramels, nut clusters, or hard candies.

Mini Gift Boxes

Mini gift boxes are ideal for a small assortment of candies and are available in holiday colors, patterns, or classic kraft paper styles. Here's how to add your touch:

- **Line with Tissue Paper**: Place a small piece of tissue paper or parchment paper inside the box for a professional look. Fold the paper over the candies to keep them in place.
- **Add a Window for Display**: If the box doesn't have a window, consider cutting a small square on the lid and covering it with clear plastic to showcase the candies inside.
- **Tie with a Ribbon**: Close the box and finish with a ribbon, twine, or lace for a polished look. Add a sprig of holly or a mini ornament for a festive touch.

Best For: Assortments of fudge, truffles, or caramels.

Reusable Jute Bags or Cotton Pouches

Eco-friendly and reusable, jute bags or cotton pouches are a unique way to gift your keto candies while providing a bonus gift bag. Here's how to make them festive:

- **Add Inner Packaging**: Place candies in small wax paper bags or cellophane inside the pouch to keep them fresh.
- **Personalize the Bag**: Use fabric markers or iron-on designs to add a holiday message, the recipient's name, or your own artwork.
- **Embellish with Greenery**: Tie a sprig of fresh rosemary or eucalyptus around the bag's drawstring for an elegant touch.

Best For: Small candies like truffles, clusters, or wrapped caramels.

Decorative Glassine or Wax Paper Bags

Glassine bags or wax paper bags have a smooth, semi-transparent finish, making them perfect for a simple, stylish presentation:

- **Fold and Seal with Stickers**: After placing the candies in the bag, fold down the top and seal it with a decorative holiday sticker or a strip of washi tape.
- **Layer Multiple Bags**: Use separate bags for each type of candy, then stack and tie them together with twine or a ribbon for a variety pack.
- **Add a Tag or Charm**: Punch a small hole in the corner of the bag and attach a tag or small charm for a personalized touch.

Best For: Fudge squares, hard candies, or brittle.

Snow Globe Candy Jars

For a truly festive gift, try creating a snow globe candy jar! This creative idea adds a holiday decoration along with the candy.

- **Layer the Candy in a Jar**: Use a small mason jar or glass container and fill it with your candy.
- **Add a Holiday Scene on the Lid**: Glue a small holiday figurine, such as a snowman, Christmas tree, or reindeer, onto the lid. Sprinkle a bit of faux snow around it for a snow globe effect.
- **Decorate the Jar**: Wrap the lid with a ribbon and add a tag with the candy's name.

Best For: Fudge, peppermint bark, or caramels.

DIY Holiday Cones

For a unique presentation, make DIY cones with decorative paper. They're perfect for small portions and create a beautiful display.

- **Roll Decorative Paper into Cones**: Use holiday-themed scrapbook paper to roll into cone shapes and secure with tape or glue.
- **Line with Parchment**: Add a small piece of parchment or wax paper inside to keep the candy from sticking.
- **Tie with a Ribbon**: Place candies in the cone, fold over the top, and tie it with a holiday ribbon.

Best For: Small candies like nut clusters, caramels, or truffles.

Holiday Themed Tinsn and Jars with Custom Labels

Holiday-themed tins and jars are perfect for gifting larger amounts of candy or assorted varieties. Personalizing the container makes the gift even more special:

- **Decorate with Custom Labels**: Design and print labels with the recipient's name, the candy type, or a holiday message. Adhesive labels work well on tins and jars.
- **Fill with Candy Variety**: Layer different types of candy for a visually appealing gift, and include a mini card describing each flavor or type.
- **Finish with Festive Ribbon and Charm**: Wrap a holiday ribbon around the container and add a small charm, bell, or decorative ornament for extra flair.

Best For: Large batches of fudge, brittle, or assorted candies.

Final Thoughts

Presenting your homemade keto candies in thoughtful, creative packaging adds a special touch that friends and family will appreciate. With a little attention to detail and some holiday-inspired decorations, you can transform your delicious creations into beautiful, memorable gifts. Each package will show the care and effort you've put into making and sharing something sweet.

Happy gifting, and enjoy the holiday cheer as you share your keto creations with loved ones!

Conclusion

As we bring this cookbook to a close, I hope you feel as excited and inspired as I do about the possibilities of a keto Christmas. The holiday season holds a special place in our hearts, a time for gathering with loved ones, sharing in laughter, and enjoying traditions that bring us comfort and joy. With the recipes and tips in this book, you've been given the tools to celebrate without compromise, savoring every delicious bite while staying true to your keto lifestyle.

From indulgent chocolate truffles to crisp, spiced nuts, this collection was designed to remind you that embracing a healthier way of eating doesn't mean sacrificing the sweetness of the season. Each recipe is crafted to deliver all the flavor and satisfaction you crave without the carb overload that traditional treats bring. I hope that you'll find new holiday favorites among these pages, ones you'll return to year after year as you celebrate the magic of Christmas.

Remember, living a keto lifestyle is more than just a way of eating—it's a commitment to honoring your body and well-being. Each low-carb treat you make is a gift to yourself, affirming your goals and the healthy choices that have brought you this far. And as you share these treats with family and friends, you're spreading that same message of mindful indulgence and festive cheer.

Thank you for allowing me to be a part of your holiday kitchen. May these recipes bring joy, flavor, and a touch of holiday magic to your celebrations. Wishing you a warm, wonderful, and *Karbvelous* keto Christmas—one filled with love, laughter, and sweet memories that linger long after the season fades.

Warm wishes,

Carolyn Boheler

About the Author

Carolyn Boheler's journey with weight and health challenges began in 1987 when she was diagnosed with Hashimoto's disease. This autoimmune condition led to the destruction of her thyroid gland through radiation, causing her to struggle with weight issues for many years. However, Carolyn found hope and success through the ketogenic lifestyle. By embracing keto, she not only managed to lose the weight but also kept it off, transforming her life in the process.

In her new book, Carolyn shares the recipes and "tricks" that have made this lifestyle sustainable and achievable. Her personal experience and practical advice offer readers a blueprint for a healthier, more fulfilling life, making the journey not just possible but enjoyable.

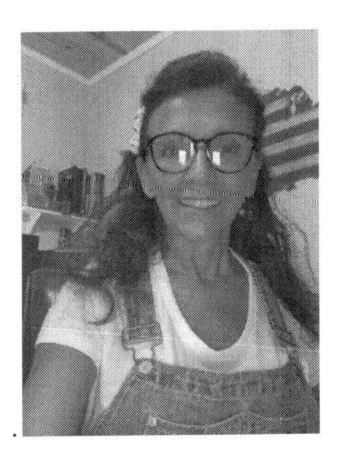

www.GoodSensePublishing.com

Karbvelous Keto

Transform Your Plate, Transform Your Life

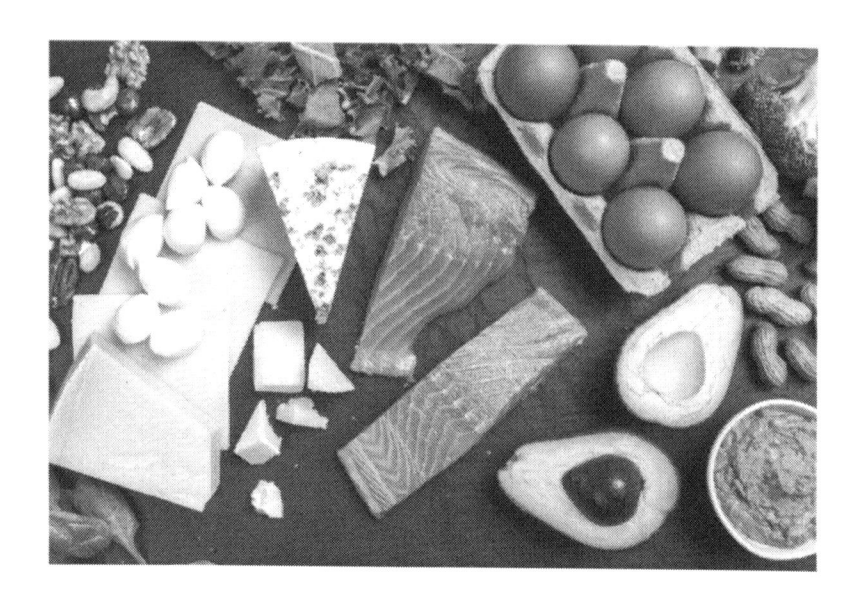

by: Carolyn Boheler, PhD

Purchase Online at : https://amzn.to/3YUJkyx

Karbvelous Keto

Transform Your Plate, Transform Your Life

Thanksgiving Edition

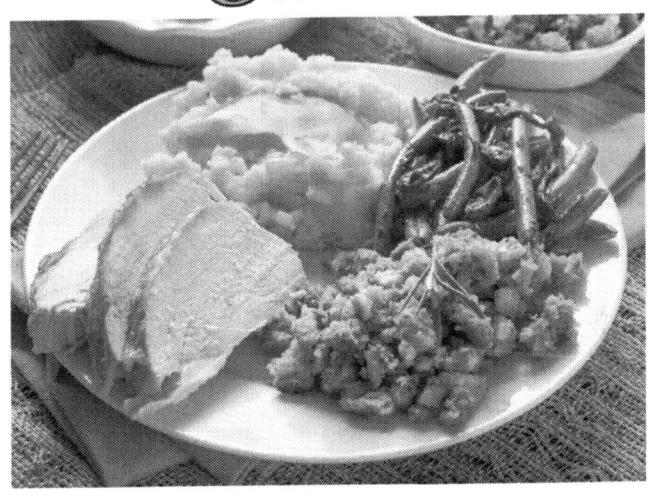

Carolyn Boheler, PhD

Purchase Online at : https://amzn.to/4fEp2yR

Books by my Mother

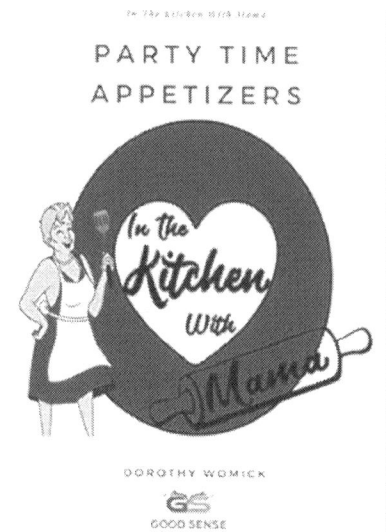

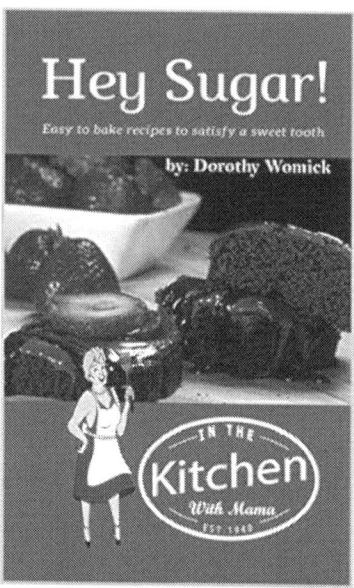

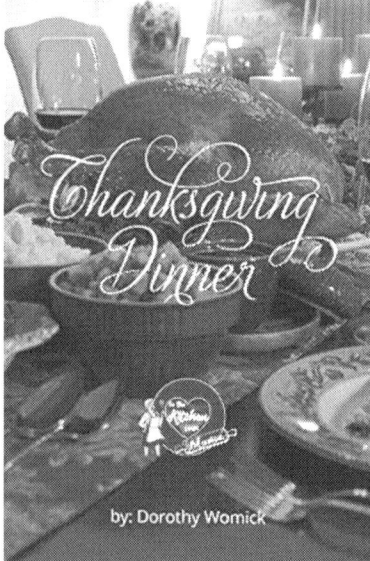

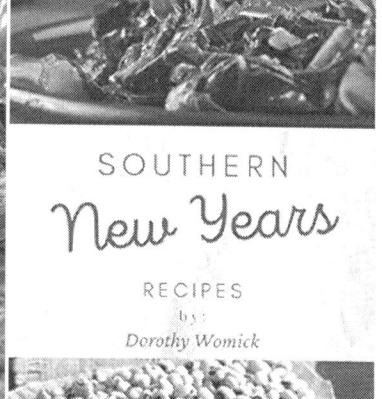

Available online at https://GoodSensePublishing.com

Acknowledgments

This book would not have been possible without the support and encouragement of many people. First and foremost, I want to thank my family and friends for their unwavering belief in me, even when the journey seemed long and difficult. Your love and support have been my greatest motivation.

To my medical team, thank you for your guidance and care over the years. Your expertise helped me navigate the challenges of Hashimoto's disease, and I am deeply grateful for your dedication to my health and well-being.

I also want to express my gratitude to the community, both online and offline, for sharing their experiences, tips, and encouragement. You have shown me that I am not alone on this journey, and your stories have inspired me to keep going.

A special thank you to my readers—your interest in this book is what drives me to share my story and my recipes. I hope that what I've learned and created will help you find success and joy in your keto journey.

Finally, to everyone who has contributed to this book, whether through feedback, taste-testing, or simply cheering me on—thank you. This book is a reflection of the love, support, and knowledge that I have been fortunate to receive, and I am honored to share it with all of you.

Please take the time to leave a review if you've enjoyed my books.
https://amzn.to/3YOY1Ce

Thank you so much!

I've included links to items found on Amazon that are used in the recipes within this book. When you click one of these links, I may earn a small commission, but rest assured, your price will not be higher because of it. Occasionally, you might even find a better deal!
The links are clickable on the Kindle or ebook versions, or you can find a page of links at www.GoodSensePublishing.

Made in the USA
Columbia, SC
24 November 2024